HEALTHY JUICING FOR BEGINNERS

365+ Days of Easy and Effective Juicing Recipes Proven to Boost Weight Loss, Enhance Body Detox, Gain Energy, and Improve Wellness Overall

DoubleTree Press

© **Copyright DoubleTree Press 2021 - All rights reserved.**

The content contained within this book may not be reproduced, duplicated or transmitted without direct written permission from the author or the publisher.

Under no circumstances will any blame or legal responsibility be held against the publisher, or author, for any damages, reparation, or monetary loss due to the information contained within this book. Either directly or indirectly.

Legal Notice:

This book is copyright protected. This book is only for personal use. You cannot amend, distribute, sell, use, quote or paraphrase any part, or the content within this book, without the consent of the author or publisher.

Disclaimer Notice:

By reading this document, the reader agrees that under no circumstances is the author responsible for any losses, direct or indirect, which are incurred as a result of the use of information contained within this document, including, but not limited to, — errors, omissions, or inaccuracies.

Table of Contents

INTRODUCTION 14

CHAPTER 1: JUICING BASICS 15

   WHAT IS JUICING? 15
   TOP REASONS TO START JUICING 16
      It's an efficient way to meet your recommended daily fruit and vegetable requirements.................... 16
      Juicing cleanses and detoxifies the body 16
      Juicing is an effective stressbuster 16
      Juicing is the ultimate energy-booster 16
      Juicing improves brain function 16
      Juicing improves sleep 16
      Juicing hydrates the body 16
      Juicing builds and strengthens bones 17
      Juicing strengthens the immune system 17
      Juicing improves overall health and wellness 17
      Helps you lose pounds and maintain a healthy weight 17
      Helps improve your skin and complexion 17
      Helps to keep your blood pressure in check 17
      Helps regulate your blood sugar levels 17
      Helps improve the functions of your digestive system 17
      Helps you add a broader variety of fruits and vegetables to your diet 17
      Helps return your body to a healthy alkaline state 18
      Helps you save time and energy with meal preparation 18
      Helps you take control of your diet 18
      Helps you feel happier 18
   FINDING THE RIGHT JUICER 18
      What to Look for When Buying a Juicer 18
   THE THREE MAIN TYPES OF JUICERS 19
      Centrifugal Juicers 19
      Masticating or Single Gear Juicers 20
      Triturating or Twin Gear Juicers 21
   WHO CAN DRINK RAW JUICES AND HOW OFTEN? 22
   WHEN IS THE BEST TIME OF DAY TO DRINK YOUR JUICES? 22
   PURPOSE OF JUICING 23
      Juicing for Cleansing and Detoxification 23
      Juicing to Supplement your Diet 23
   THE MUST-HAVE TOOLS 23

- *The Juicer* 23
- *Cutting Board and Knife* 24
- *Airtight Pitcher or Mason jars* 24
- *Sink Basket* 24
- *Blender* 24
- *Top Juicing Books* 24
- *Cleaner* 24
- *Kitchen Helpers* 24
- *Supply Storage* 24

BUYING PRODUCE 25
STEPS TO MAKE YOUR JUICE 25
ENSURING BALANCED FLAVOR 25
- *Choose the Right Sweeteners* 25
- *Find the Right Formula* 26
- *Don't Be Afraid to Experiment* 26

TAKING CARE OF YOUR JUICER 26
WASHING AND PREPARING PRODUCE 27
COMMON FRUITS AND VEGGIES TO USE WHEN JUICING 27
- *Fruits* 27
- *Vegetables* 30
- *Spices* 32

STORING YOUR JUICES FOR LATER USE 33
TIPS FOR JUICING SUCCESS 34
- *Read the Manual* 34
- *Don't Overload the Juicer* 34
- *Make It Fit* 34
- *Reuse the Pulp* 34
- *Aim for Green* 34
- *Rotate Ingredients* 34
- *Choose Organic When Possible* 35
- *Adjust for Taste* 35
- *Cold Juice Tastes Best* 35
- *Freeze Fruits and Veggies* 35

CHAPTER 2: DETOXING RECIPES 36

CHARD LIME GREEN JUICE 36
ARUGULA ORANGE MINT JUICE 36
TANGY BEETY DETOX JUICE 37
SPINACH ORANGE CELERY JUICE 37
FENNEL DILL APPLE JUICE 38
APPLE STRAWBERRY SPINACH JUICE 38
GREEN DETOX JUICE 39

- Fresh Cilantro Lettuce Orange juice 39
- Coconut Pineapple Lettuce Juice 40
- Refreshing Lean Green Juice 40
- Pear Lemon Cucumber Juice 40
- Fruity Spinach Detox Juice 41
- Harmless Purple Passion Juice 41
- Dreamy Watermelon Juice 42
- Liver Cleanse Juice 42
- The Secret Pink Juice 43
- Green Goddess Detox Juice 43
- Golden Detox Juice 44
- Sweet Beet Detox Juice 44
- Super Detox Juice 45
- Citrus Beet Detox Juice 45
- The Root Detox Juice 46

CHAPTER 3 : JUICES FOR AILMENTS 47

- Fennel Fabulous Juice 47
- The Green Man Juice 47
- Sunset Juice 48
- Parsnip Juice 48
- Kale-Cium Juice 49
- Blood-Building Elixir Juice 49
- Colon Friendly Green Juice 50
- Intestine Scrubbing Pomegranate Green Juice 50
- Minty Orange Juice 51
- Creamsicle Juice 51
- Very Berry Juice 52
- Beet and Veggies Juice 52
- Green Goddess Juice 52
- Cucumber and Kale Lemonade Juice 53
- Jump Starter Juice 53
- The Red Eye Juice 54
- Hearty Spinach Juice 54
- The Oprah Green Juice 55
- Ginger and Lemon Juice 55
- Mixed Carrot Juice 56
- Alzheimer's Cure juice 56
- Sweetened Broccoli Juice 57
- Avocado Green Juice 57
- Bright Turmeric Juice 58
- Coconut Splash Juice 58

- Anti-Diabetic Greens Pear Smoothie 59
- Dragon Fruit Juice 59
- The Immune Juice 60
- Golden Beet Juice 60
- Red Peppered Juice 61
- Apple and Celery Juice 61
- Sweet Beet Juice 62
- Cashew and Strawberry Juice 62
- Peachy Immunity Juice 63

CHAPTER 4: OVERALL HEALTH AND WELLNESS RECIPES 64

- Magic Lemony Apple Juice 64
- Coco Berry Smoothie 64
- Cardiovascular Health Almond Cinnamon Smoothie 65
- Oily Citrus Smoothie 65
- The Medley of Romaine and Orange Juice 66
- Greasy Mango Smoothie 66
- Berry Pastiche Smoothie 67
- Citrus Avocado Smoothie 67
- Carrot and Sweet Lime Juice 68
- The "Ginger" First Aid Juice 68
- Radiantly Red Juice 69
- Green Celery Juice 69
- Lemon "Get Up and Go" Smoothie 70
- The "Beet Goes On" Juice 70
- Cabbage Cucumber Juice 71
- Mint Grape Apple Juice 71
- Super Delicious Fruit Juice 71
- Greenie Pear Smoothie 72
- Green Banana Smoothie 72
- Flaxseed Greens Smoothie 73
- Strawberry Greens Smoothie 73
- Enlivener Citrus Pear Smoothie 74
- Avocado Berry Smoothie 74
- Refreshing Lemon Berry Juice 75
- Passion Fruit Plum Juice 75
- Healthy Coconut Oil Green Juice 76
- Spicy Berry Juice 76
- Sweet and Spicy Mango Kale Juice 76
- Refreshing Mint Kiwi Juice 77
- Red Bell Pepper Apple Juice 77
- Supreme Spinach Juice 78

- Pure Carrot Juice 78
- Immunity Enhancer Greenie Strawberry Smoothie 79
- Mango Berry Smoothie 79
- Flaxy Banana Smoothie 80
- Berry Greens Smoothie 80
- The "Purple Yet Red" Juice 81
- Tropical Fruit Juice 81
- Healthy Homemade Juice 82
- Minted Fruit Cocktail Juice 82

CHAPTER 5: JUICES FOR MENTAL HEALTH 83

- Mango and Green Tea Juice 83
- Apple, Red Leaf Lettuce, and Cucumber Juice 83
- Cucumber and Apple Juice 84
- Papaya, Apple, and Dates Juice 84
- Apple, Kiwi, Pineapple, and Orange Juice 85
- Green Grape and Pepper Juice 85
- Strawberry Lime Juice 86
- The Mind and Eye Opener Juice 86
- Beetroot and Sweet Potato Juice 87
- Greens and Apple Juice 87
- Orange and Parsley Juice 88
- Muskmelon, Cactus, and Grape Juice 88
- Salty and Sweet Pineapple Juice 89
- Pineapple, Watermelon, and Mango Juice 89
- Brain Booster Juice 90

CHAPTER 6: JUICES FOR YOUTHFUL SKIN 91

- Red Cabbage, Ginger, and Grape Juice 91
- Cucumber, Kale and Spinach Juice 91
- Bruschetta Juice 92
- Heavy Metal Detox Juice 93
- Avocado, Spinach, and Lime Juice 93
- The Ultimate Skin Immune Booster Juice 94
- Sunset Passion Juice 95
- Best Face Forward Juice 95
- Refreshing Renewal Juice 96
- Ultimate Veggie Mix Juice 96
- The Green Cucumber Juice 97
- Pink Delight Juice 97
- Ginger Root Boost Juice 98
- Ginger-Watermelon Juice 98
- The Go-To Juice 98

- Blue Grape-fruity Juice 99
- The Belly Settler Juice 99
- Beet Cool Dude Juice 100
- Green Garlic Monster Juice 100
- Cucumber Beet Juice 101
- Dessert Juice 101
- Peach Sunrise Juice 102
- Swiss Chard and Goji Berry Juice 102
- Glowing Skin Juice 103
- Green Machine Juice 103
- Parsley Energy Juice 104
- Swiss Chard Kale Juice 104
- Kiwi Orange Juice 105
- Grape-Beet Juice 105
- Sweet Potato, Bell Pepper, Beet and Carrot Juice 106
- Asparagus, Coriander, and Onion Juice 106
- Morning Glory Juice 107
- Kale Anti-Aging Juice 107
- Mango and Pineapple Juice 108
- Broccoli and Pear Juice 108
- Carrot and Pineapple Juice 109

CHAPTER 7: JUICES FOR WEIGHT LOSS 110

- Fresh Cilantro Lettuce Orange juice 110
- Grapefruit Mint Lettuce Juice 111
- Grape Spinach Kiwi Juice 111
- Kale Powerade Juice 112
- Mexican Bell Pepper Juice 112
- Refreshing Apple Mint Juice 113
- Dandelion Parsley Kale Juice 113
- Spinach Ginger Lemon Juice 114
- Mint Watercress Beet Juice 114
- Kiwi and Cucumber Juice 115
- Carrot and Broccoli Juice 115
- Ginger Garlic Green Juice 116
- Green Juice for Healthy Eye 116
- Melon and Wheatgrass Juice 117
- Watercress and Apple Juice 117
- Lemony Grapefruit Juice 118
- Citrus Mango Juice 118
- Simple Nice Green Juice 119
- "Kitchen Sink" Detox Juice 119

Crazy Cabbage Juice 120
Citrus Weight Buster Juice 120
Sparkling Health Drink Juice 121
Weight Loss Tonic Juice 121
Apple Cucumber Basil Juice 122
Parsley Lime Pineapple Juice 122
Apple Pear Swiss chard Juice 123
Coconut Pineapple Lettuce Juice 123
Chard Lime Green Juice 124
Refreshing Lean Green Juice 124
Cool as a Cucumber Juice 125
Cinnamon Circulation Booster Juice 125
Antioxidant Bok Choy Juice 126
Low Cal Tropical Punch Juice 126
Berry Super Lunch Juice 127
Hungry Orange Crush Juice 127
Citrus and Mango Love Juice 128
Pear Lemon Cucumber Juice 128
Watercress Cucumber Blackberry Green Juice 129
Lettuce Ginger Carrot Juice 129
Spinach Orange Celery Juice 130
Fennel Dill Apple Juice 130
Apple Strawberry Spinach Juice 131
The Weight Loss Bunny Brew Juice 131
The Cool Pink Pom Juice 132
The Mean Belly Buster Juice 132
The Cellulite Fat Killer Juice 133

CHAPTER 8: JUICES FOR ENERGY BOOSTING 134

Brussels Green Juice 134
Green Pumpkin Smoothie 134
Seven Green Giant Layers Juice 135
Breezy Green Juice 135
Whole Green Goodness Juice 136
Ginger Pear Juice 136
Apple Basil Kiwi Juice 137
Cranberry Pomegranate Juice 137
Energy Booster Green Juice 138
Green Peach Drink Juice 138
Coconut and Litchi Juice 139
Goji Berry Juice 139
Wheatgrass Carrot Juice 140

Avocado Sprout Smoothie 140
Energizer Juice 141
Strawberry and Apple Juice 141
Beet Martini Juice 142
Cabbage Patch Juice 142
Cognition Booster Juice 143
Cilantro Apple Green Juice 143
Pineapple Cucumber Kale Juice 144
Banana Berry Smoothie 144
Energizing Purple Juice 145
Masterpiece of Green Goodness Juice 145
Amazing Sunflower Greens Smoothie 146
Green Tango Juice 146
Energetic Litchi Blueberry Juice 147
Morning Buzz Juice 147
Hot Green Lover Juice 148
Pineapple, Banana, and Kale Smoothie 148
Ginger Power Smoothie 149
Green Dream Juice 149
Green Avocado Smoothie 150
Berry Cauliflower Smoothie 150
Pineapple Wheatgrass Smoothie 151
Holy Kale Cleanse Juice 151
Very Berry Smoothie 152
Green Dawn Juice 152
Grape Dates Green Smoothie 153
Power Jumble Smoothie 153
Three C's Juice 154
Spicy Orange Surprise Juice 154
Blood Orange Juice 155
Purple Passion Juice 155
The Green Clean Pineapple Juice 156
Lime and Honeydew Melon Juice 156
Pear Juice 156

CONCLUSION 158

Introduction

Juicing fruits and vegetables has a positive effect on your overall health and lifestyle. Take charge by incorporating these delicious healthy juicing blends into your daily diet instead of avoiding various fruits and vegetables. This book is a reference book; you can continuously refer to the health benefits of these various fruits and vegetables and choose a different juice blend each day. I encourage you to write a food journal consisting of the whole foods and juicing blends that you ingest. Within this journal, describe how you feel at the end of each day and see if the addition of fresh juice makes a positive difference in your life. Remember to change the type of juice blend you drink each day, so you are able to receive all the health benefits that these delicious refreshing juices have to offer.

Juicing can help feed your body with the essential vitamins and minerals it needs while helping you to lose weight healthily. That is exactly what I hope to teach you throughout the pages of this recipe book. Throughout this book, not only do I hope you discover the best ingredients to add to your homemade juice recipes, but that you feel encouraged to try new juicing recipes in the process. By the end of this book, I know you will want to make as many healthy juices as often as possible. So, let's stop wasting time and get to juicing!

Chapter 1: Juicing Basics

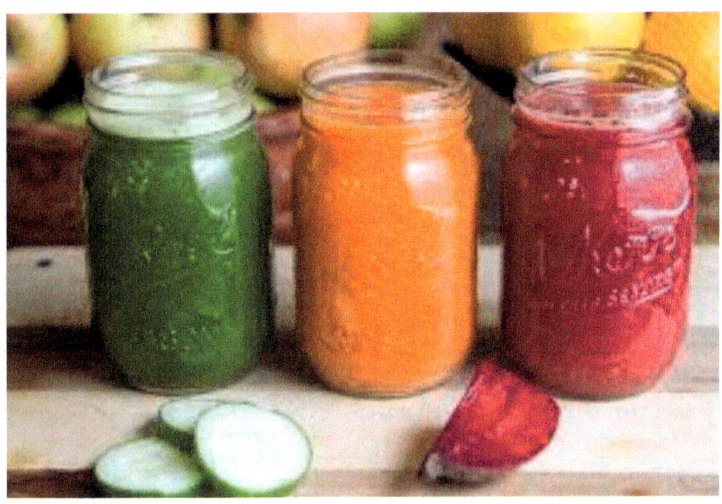

What Is Juicing?

Juicing is basically a process of extracting the liquid content of raw veggies and fruits. What the process of juicing does is that it segregates and gets rid of the solid matter of the vegetables and fruits which includes the seeds, skin, and pulp, and retains the liquid juice for consumption. This juice is packed with vitamins, minerals, phytonutrients, antioxidants, and other nutrients in its complete natural state.

Juicing is an enjoyable yet efficient way to consume a variety of fruits and vegetables while gaining the maximum benefit of the vitamins, minerals, and other important nutrients they contain. And because the juice is in liquid form, your body can utilize these essential nutrients much faster than when you eat fruits and vegetables prepared in the traditional way.

Many people often mistake juicing with blending. While both methods have proven to be beneficial to health when done consistently, the two concepts are different.

Juicers produce fresh juice by separating the produce's fiber and liquid. On the other hand, blending makes use of a blender to produce a smoothie that contains both the juice and the fiber of the produce. With juicing, you end up with a pure juice or a blend of juices, depending on the ingredients you choose. With blending, the produce is pureed, usually with other ingredients such as milk, yogurt, sweeteners, nuts, seeds, water, and more.

Because the fiber of the fruits and vegetables are retained with blending, many people think that it is the healthier method of the two. The truth is that although fresh juices lack fiber, they are more nutrient-dense compared to smoothies.

A glass of juice makes use of more fruits and vegetables compared to a glass of smoothie, helping you get more nutrition in a smaller package. With the fiber and pulp out of the way with a glass of fresh juice, you will get more nutrition with less volume

Top Reasons to Start Juicing

People go into juicing for a variety of reasons. Some do it to lose weight, to detox, or to simply start a healthy lifestyle. Whatever your reason, here are a few more reasons why juicing is the best decision you'll ever make for your body.

It's an efficient way to meet your recommended daily fruit and vegetable requirements

Let's face it, if you were to choose between a plateful of veggies or a slice of cake, you'd choose the latter in a heartbeat. This is where juicing comes in – even if you're not a fan of fruits and vegetables (or not all of them), it's a fun and easy way to consume your daily quota of produce in just one glass.

Juicing cleanses and detoxifies the body

We are exposed to thousands and thousands of harmful toxins everyday which can lead to a variety of health problems. Juicing can help rid your system of these toxins and also cleanse your body of disease-causing bacteria, keeping you in tip-top shape.

Juicing is an effective stressbuster

Because juicing can help you get a variety of essential nutrients from different fruits and vegetables, it helps prevent many health threats such as excess stress. Important nutrients such as Vitamin C and magnesium help control the stress hormone cortisol.

Juicing is the ultimate energy-booster

You need energy to face all of life's daily demands. And because juice is in liquid form, you are able to absorb the nutrients from different produce almost instantly. Because of this, your body doesn't require extra energy to break down food, leaving you with more energy to use for other activities.

Juicing improves brain function

Juicing increases blood flow to the brain, which helps it to function better and decreases the risk of cognitive decline and dementia.

Juicing improves sleep

Fresh juice recipes often make use of green leafy vegetables which are rich in magnesium, a mineral proven to help the body relax, therefore making it easier to sleep.

Juicing hydrates the body

Fresh fruit and vegetable juices are often referred to as "nature's vitamin water." Like water, a glass of fresh juice quenches thirst and rejuvenates the body while providing it with essential vitamins and minerals.

Juicing builds and strengthens bones

Vegetables such as broccoli, collard greens, and kale, which are often used in green juices, are good sources of calcium and magnesium. These two minerals are vital for bone-building and strengthening.

Juicing strengthens the immune system

The antioxidants and other essential nutrients in fresh juice help fight health problems caused by fatty and processed food, reducing the risk of diseases like cancer, diabetes, and heart disease.

Juicing improves overall health and wellness

By regularly drinking fresh fruit and vegetable juices, you will become more energized and better able to handle stress – and therefore happier and healthier.

Helps you lose pounds and maintain a healthy weight

Many people go into juicing for its weight-loss benefits. Because fruits and vegetables are high in fiber, fresh juices make you feel full longer, helping you to avoid overeating.

Helps improve your skin and complexion

Juicing helps flush out toxins, hydrates the skin, and protects it from free radicals. As a result, you will have a healthier, smoother, and more radiant complexion.

Helps to keep your blood pressure in check

Foods that are low in sodium like fruits and vegetables help lower blood pressure. And because juicing helps reduce weight, that also helps decrease blood pressure.

Helps regulate your blood sugar levels

When you choose your fruits carefully or use a minimal number of fruits high in fructose, fresh fruit and vegetable juices have a low natural sugar content, which helps maintain healthy blood sugar levels.

Helps improve the functions of your digestive system

Because raw juices require little digestion, your digestive tract is able to rest when you drink juice. The potent nutrients from the juice also nourish the different systems in your body, including your digestive system.

Helps you add a broader variety of fruits and vegetables to your diet

When you eat fruits and vegetables, most likely you only eat the ones you like. With juicing, you will be able to consume a wider variety of produce with different colors and get the specific nutrients each of them contains.

Helps return your body to a healthy alkaline state

Unhealthy foods mess with your blood's pH balance, which can lead to health problems. Juicing can help minimize the acidic effects of unhealthy foods and bring back your body's healthy pH levels.

Helps you save time and energy with meal preparation

One way to stay healthy is to cook nutritious home-cooked meals and avoid fast food. But not all of us have time to prepare 3 balanced meals a day, so juicing is a good way to stay healthy – just throw your ingredients in a juicer and you're good to go!

Helps you take control of your diet

With juicing, you have the freedom to be creative with your diet – you can mix and match the produce you want and play with different tastes and textures.

Helps you feel happier

Juicing makes you more energized and refreshed, leading to a healthier, happier life.

Finding the Right Juicer

One of the most important yet often overlooked elements of juicing is finding the right juicer to use. The most important advice I can give you regarding this is to look for a juicer that best works for you. Different juicers cater to different needs; what's important is to purchase one that best meets your personal needs.

There are many different varieties of juicers on the market today which makes it difficult for a beginner like you to choose one. When buying a juicer, it is important that you consider factors such as availability, performance, and price. For a better juicing experience, weigh your options carefully before deciding on what type of juicer to buy.

What to Look for When Buying a Juicer

Ease of Operation

As a beginner, it's helpful to buy a juicer that is easy to set up, use, and clean afterward.

Quality of Juice

Some juicers work by smashing the produce, breaking down some of its beneficial chemicals. Choose a juicer that will give you quality juice – one that has high enzyme and nutrient content. Some juicers also spin very fast, producing juice that has a higher oxidation rate, which makes it spoil faster. Balance these factors and buy an efficient machine that gives you good, quality juice.

Power and Speed

For a beginner, a juicer that has at least 1/4 horsepower would be good enough. Cheaper machines usually have less power which tends to give you lower quality juice. Another thing to consider is speed. The faster your juicer works, the more time you save.

Yield Per Pound

Cheaper juicers make less juice out of your fruit and vegetables compared to higher quality ones. Choose a juicer that is reasonably priced but gives you up to 25% more juice compared to cheaper models.

Lasting Power

Cheaper models of juicers (priced less than $100) come with low-quality motors which may wear out easily because they can't handle cores, rinds, and seeds. Go for a higher-priced juicer if you can (in the $200-$300 price range). Remember, you get what you pay for.

The Three Main Types of Juicers

There are three main types of juicers: Centrifugal, Masticating, and Triturating Juicers. Each of these juicers has pros and cons which need to be weighed carefully in order to choose the perfect juicer for your needs.

Centrifugal Juicers

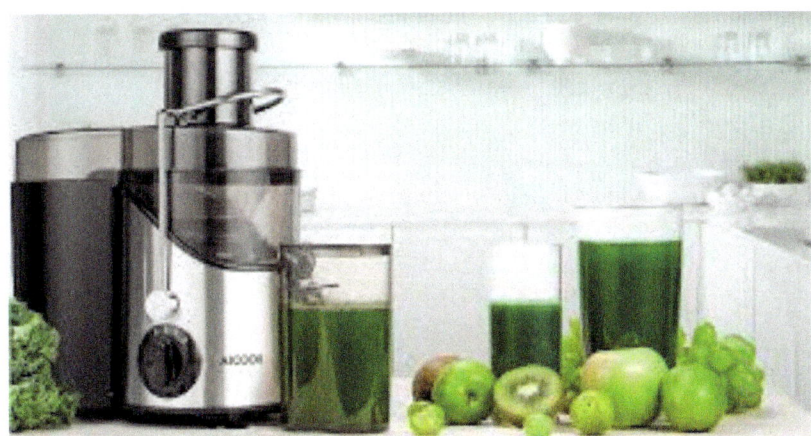

Centrifugal juicers are among the popular choices in juicers. They are recommended for beginners and those who are on a budget.

They have a fast, rotating blade that provides centrifugal force, shredding the produce instantly and ejecting the pulp into a container.

Pros:

- Affordable

- Easy to clean

- Works fast

- Usually has a large opening, so there's less work for cutting and preparing vegetables

- Good for juicing most soft fruits and hard-root vegetables

Cons:

- Loud

- Extracts less juice from pulp compared to more expensive models

- Fast action may result in foaming and oxidation of the juice

- Not ideal for juicing leafy greens

Masticating or Single Gear Juicers

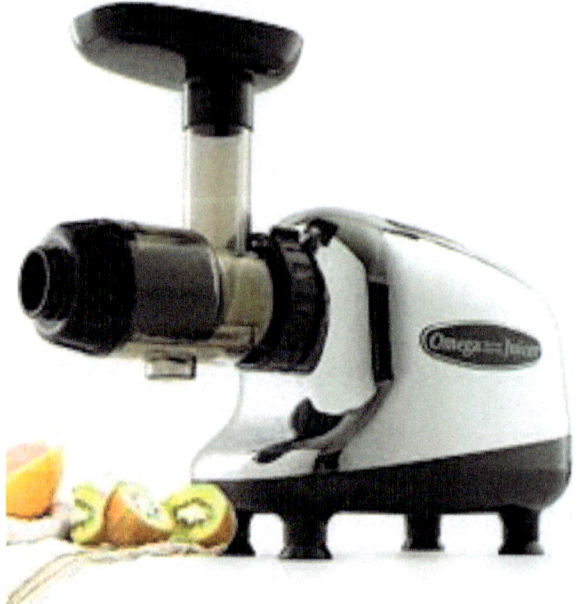

Also called the "single auger juicer", this machine can crush and grind a larger variety of fruits and vegetables, leafy greens, and even nuts. It works by crushing the produce, extracting the pulp into a container before squeezing out the juice. Some people also use it as a food processor because it can mince nuts and vegetables.

Pros:

- Easiest to clean among all types of juicers
- Ideal for juicing almost all kinds of vegetables including leafy greens
- Produces a drier pulp, which means it extracts more nutrients from the produce
- Can be used as a food processor to make sauces, nut butters, baby food, sorbet, etc.
- Operates more quietly than centrifugal juicers
- Durable, usually comes with a 10-year plus warranty

Cons:

- Works slower compared to centrifugal juicers
- Not ideal to use for juicing soft fruits
- Has a smaller opening which means more work preparing the produce
- Takes up the most counter space among all types of juicers
-

Triturating or Twin Gear Juicers

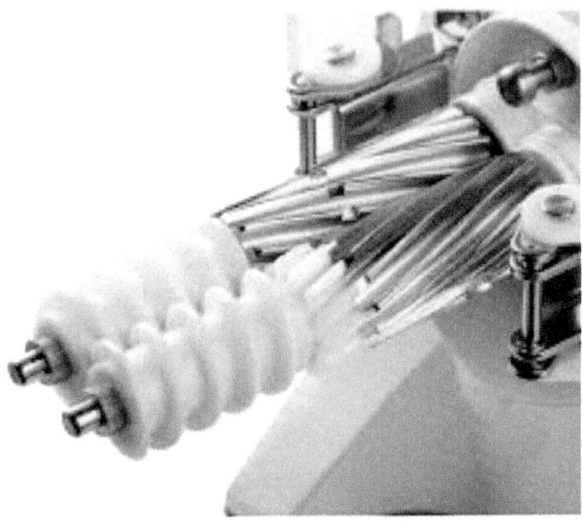

The triturating juicer is a favorite among expert juicers because of the machine's versatility. It operates similarly to the masticating juicer but is more efficient. This high-end juicer is equipped with two interlocking screws that work together to crush and grind produce.

Pros:

- Excellent at juicing any type of produce – both soft and hard fruits and vegetables, leafy greens, and nuts
- Produces the driest pulp and gives the most high-quality juice
- Can also double as a food processor which can make sauces, nut butters, baby food, sorbet, etc.
- Usually in an upright design which takes up less counter space

Cons:

- The most expensive among all types of juicers
- The hardest to clean among all types of juicers

Who Can Drink Raw Juices and How Often?

Juicing is for everyone! Anyone who wants to start eating clean or to have a healthier lifestyle can try juicing. Just be sure to check in with your health professional before you try any dietary changes, especially if you plan to undergo a juice fast.

During a juice fast or juice cleanse, you basically consume just raw juices as meal replacements for an extended period of time. This is performed mostly for detoxification purposes – to flush out toxins from your system and to give your body time to rest from performing metabolic processes.

Beginners are advised to go through an initial 1-2 days of juice fast to help prepare their bodies for the change in diet. However, if you simply want to eat healthier and add a variety of fruits and vegetables to your diet through juicing, drink a glass or two of raw juice per day in addition to your regular meals.

When Is the Best Time of Day to Drink Your Juices?

While drinking a glass of fresh fruit or vegetable juice is beneficial any time of the day, the best time to have a glass is during the morning, on an empty stomach. This way, your body can absorb the nutrients easily and you will be energized for the rest of the day.

If you plan to drink a glass of fresh juice later in the day, do it at least an hour before a meal. If you plan to drink it with a meal, be sure that the meal is light and that you drink the juice slowly.

Drinking fresh juice in the evening is beneficial as well – I usually drink a glass an hour or two before bedtime or after an evening workout to rehydrate my body.

Purpose of Juicing

Juicing for Cleansing and Detoxification

With the lifestyle and diet today, your bodies are stuffed with toxins.

Fresh fruit juice and vegetable juice diet are the best way to cleanse and detoxify your body. Cleansing your body using juices has an advantage in the fact that it avoids the stress of digesting solid food even when providing the essential nutrients to your body.

There are a number of fresh juices that can be made for flushing out the toxins and free radicals from your body. Your liver, your kidneys, and your colon are the main detoxifying organs, and hence juicing to cleanse these organs only results in improved health and vitality.

Juicing for cleansing and detoxification include juices that help in re-inoculating the detox-organs with good bacteria and at the same time soothing them of any pain or inflammation.

Juicing to Supplement your Diet

With this fast-paced life, many of you are skipping meals and eating unhealthily. Most of you are losing the essential nutrients required by the body to maintain good health.

At times you are unable to consume the recommended veggies and fruits per day. A glass of juice can supplement the nutrients that are lacking. Juices are a quick way for the body to assimilate the necessary vitamins, minerals, and other nutrients as it is in the soluble form.

Juices can help to replenish and nourish your body but remember that juices are supplements to whole foods and cannot be made a replacement.

The Must-Have Tools

By now you should have an idea that juicing is more than simply blending the fruits and veggies! It is more of a form of art. And just like any other form of art, you are going to need several different things to ensure that you can enjoy your juicing journey fully.

The Juicer

At the very heart of any juicing environment, lies the core of the package that is the Juicer itself! There are a wide variety of Juicers available in the market and each of them has its own unique twist when it comes to juicing. I will give you all the information that you will need before choosing your perfect Juicer momentarily.

Cutting Board and Knife

Before juicing, you will need to chop the giant veggies and fruits into chunks. Hence having a good cutting board and a sharp knife is essential.

Airtight Pitcher or Mason jars

Once you have juiced, you should avoid it from being exposed to air for a long time. So, in case you have juiced and want to store it for a couple of hours then an airtight pitcher or a sealable mason jar is an important tool.

Sink Basket

This is of great help to wash and drain your veggies and fruits well before juicing them.

Blender

You must be thinking "now, if I already have a juicer, why even bother for a blender?" Well, it turns out that the blender fulfills the void that is left while using a Juicer. A void of not being able to enjoy the fibers and flesh of the fruits and vegetables. When you are using a juicer, the juice is essentially separated from the flesh leaving behind the fibers as residue. On the other hand, blenders will allow you to get the benefits from both the juice and the fibers as well! The only drawback is that the taste might seem just a tiny bit underwhelming when compared with that of a juicer.

Top Juicing Books

Needless to say, if you are going to explore the world of juicing, you are going to need to have a good library of recipes to choose from. Sure, you can go ahead and browse the web, but having a complete compilation of all your favorite recipes in one place is much more convenient. That is why you purchased this book in the first place isn't it?

Cleaner

Of course, you don't want to eat bacteria-infested food. Cleaning is a very essential part of any juicing kitchen and it is a must that you have some quality cleaners to ensure that your ingredients are free of germs, dirt, and pesticides.

Kitchen Helpers

This category includes every little or big kind of kitchen appliance that might help you to make your juicing life a bit easier. For example, getting peelers to scrape off the skin of apples or cucumber, or perhaps a strawberry stem remover to easily cut your strawberry stems, thereby saving a great deal of time for you!

Supply Storage

Now, you would not want your ingredients and products to take up space all over the floor and counters; you are going to need to have an ample supply of storage boxes to make sure that your accessories and food products are kept safely in a well-organized fashion for efficient use.

Buying Produce

Just like most recipes, juice benefits from fresh, high-quality ingredients which boost flavor and nutritional content. If possible, shop at a local farmers' market where produce is fresh and has traveled a short distance from farm to market. Also, get to know the people who work at your local grocery store's produce section—they're a terrific resource for getting the inside scoop on what's in season, what's new and fresh, or what has arrived that day.

Seasonal produce is usually the most nutritious and least expensive option because there is currently an abundance being harvested. No matter the variety, look for produce that is heavy for its size, vibrant in color, and free of insect damage. Make sure the outer area is not shriveled, wrinkled, or bruised.

Steps to Make Your Juice

Making your own juice is a healthy choice. Here are the steps for your reference to prepare your own juice:

- Select the ingredients you want to use in your juice.
- Wash the ingredients well.
- Chop the ingredients to fit into your juicer.
- Feed the vegetables and fruits through your juicer, selecting the appropriate speed: high for hard produce, low for soft produce.
- Re-juice the extracted pulp in case it is still damp.
- Your juice is ready!
-

Ensuring Balanced Flavor

As we have mentioned earlier, it is important to prepare and accustom yourself to the tastes and flavors of various combinations of fruits and vegetables. Juicing is not just about simply extracting juice from produce. This is also about being able to maximize the health benefits of juicing without sacrificing taste and flavor.

At the same time, finding the right balance of fruits and vegetables—in terms of variants and quantities—is not just a fun process, it will also ultimately determine whether juicing can become an integral part of your dietary habits.

Choose the Right Sweeteners

If you need to sweeten your juice but do not like to use carrots, then you can add apples instead.

Specifically, Granny Smith apples are best for this purpose because they are not so sweet, a little bit sour, and better able to complement the flavors of extracted vegetable juice.

To balance the flavor, you can also add some lime or lemon juice so that the juice can also have a refreshing and cleansing function. The acidity of citrus juices can also induce healthy BM in the morning.

Find the Right Formula

Juicing is supposed to be a fun activity, not to mention a beneficial feature of anyone's diet program when properly followed. Some experts say that a good juice contains some or all the following flavors: sweetness, a tart taste, an earthy taste, a refreshing twist, and some hint of herbs and spices. Part of the fun of juicing is finding the right mix of flavors that you can incorporate into your juicing program.

Don't Be Afraid to Experiment

There is no bible as to what the right combination is to achieve the best nutrient content and flavor. At best, all we can offer are just suggestions. In the end, it's still up to you because it will be your body that's going to determine whether something is right or is not right for you.

Just remember, don't start right away with the heavy-duty, hardcore juicing staples (such as kale) if you have not yet grown accustomed to their taste. There is nothing wrong with starting with familiar fruits and vegetables, such as apples, tomatoes, kiwis, and so on.

If the juice is a bit bitter, you can add more apple slices; if the juice is too sweet, then add lime to give it an extra zing! Don't be afraid to experiment, this is the only way that you can find the perfect combination that suits you.

Taking Care of Your Juicer

Every home appliance that is used frequently experiences wear and tear. If you want to make your juicer last for as long as possible then you need to respect its limitations, size, quirks, keep it in good working order and keep it clean as well. It is always better to be safe than sorry when dealing with machinery that has sharp blades and motors.

Here are a few tips and trade secrets to ensure smooth juicing:

- Carefully wash all the produce before juicing. Remove mold, bruises, dings, and blemishes.

- Go organic whenever possible. Organic produce is certainly more expensive, but it also means you don't have to peel everything before placing the produce into the juicer and lose out on the good nutrients. Non-organic produce is sprayed with pesticides that penetrate the skins, which is the largest source of nutrients in the produce.

- Always make sure you peel tangerines, oranges, bananas, pineapples, kiwifruits, and grapefruits, even if they are organic.

- The leaves and stems of many fruits, such as small grape stems, strawberry caps, beet stems, and leaves, contain a higher concentration of nutrients. So, it is best not to take them all out.
- Cut most of the produce into sections and strips that can easily fit into your juicer tube without having to jam or force them in. Of course, with experience, you will learn what size works best.
- To catch the pulp during juicing, make sure you insert a grocery store-sized plastic bag in the pulp receptacle of your juicer. The pulp can be used for composting or cooking or can just be thrown away.

Washing and Preparing Produce

Sure, buying organic produce is a great way to avoid ingesting chemicals such as pesticides, herbicides, or synthetic fertilizers. However, it's still really important to wash all fruits and vegetables before juicing. Even organic produce contains natural microbes and bacteria on the surface. I'm sorry for this visual, but just think how many people may have handled that bunch of kale before you put it in your cart!

To streamline the process, you can do a little prep as soon as you get home from the store, such as removing the excess parts that you don't plan to juice, like radish or carrot greens, and brushing off any obvious dirt. To prevent premature wilting, save the actual rinsing of the produce until right before you juice. Also, even if you wash produce and then store it in the refrigerator, bacteria can still grow. Use a good, clean scrub brush on any produce tough enough to handle it. For softer produce, toss it in a large bowl of clean water and use your fingers to get water into all the nooks and crannies—this technique works well on foods such as kale, romaine, and blueberries. Empty the produce into a strainer and run some more water over it. You can also add about 1 cup of vinegar to every 3 cups of water in your rinse bowl, which may help kill bacteria.

Common Fruits and Veggies to Use When Juicing

<u>Fruits</u>

Apple

There is a large variety of apples and choosing from one of them greatly depends on the preference of the juicer; examples include Fuji, Granny Smith, and Golden Delicious. But the main reason you should keep an eye out for apples is that they are packed with antioxidants, dietary fiber, and flavonoids that make them very strong agents against cancer, diabetes, and other severe heart symptoms.

Apricots

Originating from Northern China, apricots are considered to be a very substantial source of vitamin A, potassium, and iron.

Asian Pears

As the name suggests, Asian Pears originate from ancient Asia and are said to be the ancestral version of all the pears that we have familiarized ourselves with today. A single pear holds up to 11% of the level of vitamin C that is generally recommended to be taken every day.

Banana

While bananas are not ideal for fruit juices due to their extremely soft texture, they are still very good sources of vitamins A, B, and C as well as B2, while also adding a fresh flavor to your juice.

Blueberries

Blueberries are the second most popular berry in the United States, and for good reason! These berries are all in all excellent sources of vitamin C and hold a large amount of fiber.

Cherries

Cherries tend to add a delicious sweetness to your juices, while at the same time being a good source of Vitamin C and fiber.

Grapefruit

Originating from the 1800s, seedless grapes and pink seedless grapefruit are known for their exceptionally savory-sweet flavor and richness in vitamin C and fiber.

Lemon

Cultivated in India for the last 2500 years, lemons are known for their smooth and rugged skin texture and abundance of vitamin C.

Lime

While lemons come from India, these little aromatic fruits come from the West Indies and Mexico! These are also abundant in vitamin C, but unlike lemon, these are much less acidic.

Oranges

Fresh oranges are mostly grown alongside the regions of Florida, California, and Arizona.

These are annual fruits and can be found all throughout the year. Oranges are widely known for their high vitamin C contents. Variations include blood oranges, navel oranges, and Valencia oranges.

Tangerine

Tangerines, alternatively called mandarins, are a close relative of oranges. They look similar in texture and boast a sweet flavor with puffy skin. They are rich in vitamins A and C alongside potassium and folate particles.

Cranberries

These are small, round-shaped fruits with a ruby-like color that grow in the marshes and bogs of Northern Europe. These are very rich in vitamin K, C, and A while helping in tackling kidney diseases.

Grapes

These fruits contain a very powerful antioxidant known as polyphenol, which helps in the long run to slow down or even prevent a multitude of cancers such as lung, mouth, and colon cancers.

Kiwifruit

These soft and fleshy fruits originating from Thailand are widely known for their vitamin K and vitamin C contents. But they are also good at supplying other minerals such as copper and a good amount of dietary fiber.

Mango

Cultivated in India, mangoes boast a huge number of benefits ranging from prevention of cancer, decrease in cholesterol levels, improving eyesight, as well as promoting a much healthier sex life.

Melons

Melons contain a good amount of vitamin C and vitamin A in the form of carotenoids as well as potassium, and a range of B complex vitamins that is basically like cherries topped with extra magnesium and fiber contents.

Papaya

Papayas are identified by their smooth and greenish-yellow colored skin. They provide a very delicious flavor that is jam-packed with carotene, flavonoids, vitamin C, pantothenic acid, and various other minerals, including potassium, magnesium, and copper.

Passion Fruit

A fruit that looks like an egg with a pretty thick and hard skin that envelopes a jelly-like golden flesh, these fruits are rich in fiber, the pulp and seeds alone contain 25 grams of fiber! The flesh houses water-soluble antioxidants and vitamin C.

Peaches

Peaches are generally regarded as being treasure troves of minerals that range from iron, manganese, magnesium, zinc, and copper. These are low-calorie fruits with no cholesterol or saturated fat!

Pineapple

A native of Central and Southern America, these discoveries of Christopher Columbus are a rich source of vitamin C! But that's not all; it also encapsulates various other benefits for the human body that includes enhancing the immune system, aiding in digestion, and increasing eye health.

Vegetables

Asparagus

The asparagus comes from the Mediterranean area of Southern Europe and has been around for more than 300 years. This is a vegetable from the lily family, and it is jam-packed with a myriad of health benefits! It is a very good source of fiber for starters, and it is also overflowing with vitamins A, E, C, and K, as well traces of important minerals.

Beet

The importance of beet in the world of juicing cannot be stressed enough. Beets are packed with iron, calcium as well as vitamin A. But that's not all, beet juices are extremely effective when it comes to getting rid of the toxins of the body and cleansing the blood.

Broccoli

A vegetable mostly popularized in the US by Italian immigrants, broccolis are good sources of pantothenic acid, dietary fiber, vitamin E, vitamin A, potassium, and a lot of other essential vitamins and minerals.

Brussels Sprouts

These are vegetables hailing from the cruciferous family and are closely related to cabbages and cauliflower. These act as a great source of vitamin B6, potassium, iron, riboflavin, and a host of other goodies.

Cabbage

One of the most ancient leafy plants, cabbage has its roots (literally) planted at the native villages of England and France from where it has now spread in both numbers and popularity. These are mostly famous for their antioxidant related benefits and as an extremely good source of vitamin C.

Carrot

Many of you might not know, but carrots originate from Afghanistan and they have been cultivated in the Mediterranean area since 500 B.C. Carrots are mostly known for their nutritional characteristics that help to protect and improve your eyesight, defend the body against various bacteria, viruses, free radical damage and inflammation and protection against cancer.

Cucumber

Dating back to ancient Babylonian times, cucumbers are often regarded as being the oldest cultivated crop known to mankind. Aside from helping in digestion, cucumbers are very well packed with a complex of B vitamins such as B5, B1, and B7, which help to control anxiety and stress.

Fennel

Fennel is well known for its fiber and folate content, but it is also an essential vegetable for its contribution of phytonutrients and ability to dial down the cholesterol level of blood.

Garlic

Garlic plays a huge role in keeping the body healthy specifically thanks to its impressive attribute of controlling the level of cholesterol in the body by increasing HDL and decreasing LDL levels. This has a direct positive effect on the heart. While the Greeks disliked it, this was a star among the Europeans.

Ginger

This is a reedy and herbaceous plant that comes in the form of a rootstock and is considered widely to be an Indian produce. Ginger has been used throughout history for its ability to relieve digestive ailments and tackle nausea, motion sickness, and even pain.

Jicama

Often pronounced as hik'-ka-ma, this vegetable is a leguminous one with an extremely large tuberous root. The addition of jicama to your juices will immediately increase the potency of the juice thanks to jicama's unique mixture of vitamins and minerals coupled with phytonutrients and organic compounds such as vitamin C, folate, vitamin B6, manganese, and other essential minerals such as copper.

Kale

This vegetable primarily flourishes during the winter season and is very much known for its similarity to cabbages with the exception of its leaves having much more curls. Kale is often used as both an animal feed as well as human food as it is packed with vitamin A, C, and good amounts of vitamin B.

Lettuce

This is a vegetable that pre-dates back to 500 B.C. during the Persian age. Thanks to its sweet and juicy nature, lettuce has been long used as a good ingredient of various kinds of salads and it is an excellent source of vitamin A, C, B, and E, with trace amounts of essential minerals of magnesium, iron, and calcium.

Parsley

This is a deviated member of the carrot family that is believed to have been cultivated during the early years of Sardinia and Italy. Parsley is packed with lots of essential vitamins including C, K, A, and B12. This vegetable helps to strengthen your immune system while fortifying your bones at the same time.

Pepper

Almost a staple product of Mexico, bell peppers were introduced through the escapades of 15th-century Spanish explorers.

Spinach

This vegetable was cultivated long before the Christian era by Greeks and Romans, and highly celebrated by the fictional sailor man Popeye! The leaves of spinach are highly concentrated with lots of vitamins such as B, A, C, E, and K alongside phosphorus, iron, and fiber as essential minerals.

String Beans

These are often referred to as Snap Beans and are basically the early pods of kidney beans. They are very good sources of molybdenum! They are also extremely potent sources of folate, copper, and dietary fiber as well as being packed with a generous amount of protein!

Tomatoes

These bubbly, red-colored fruits of Peru are often categorized as being vegetables mainly because of the way they are served to people. These are wells of nutrients and vitamins with substantial amounts of vitamin A, K, C, and a complex of vitamin B6.

Yams and Sweet Potatoes

While these two are different in nature, they are still often mistaken for having the same type of size and texture. These are high in vitamin C and A and contain good amounts of fiber and potassium.

Wheatgrass

Wheatgrass comes from the red wheat berry and is a special grass strain that has a very high concentration of vitamins, chlorophyll, vitamins, and activated enzymes amongst other nutrients and minerals. These include phosphorus, magnesium, iron, potassium, the whole vitamin B complex, and vitamin E, C, and K.

Spices

Cayenne Pepper

If you can survive the intense spicy flavor, then cayenne pepper can be used as a very strong anti-allergen and antifungal agent to thoroughly clear up stomach problems, sore throats due to cough, ulcers, and even severe cases of diarrhea.

Turmeric

The yellow spice mostly known as turmeric is boasted for its positive effects on the body's immune system. It helps to fortify the system as well as improve the conditions of the cardiovascular system and prevent the development of cancerous cells.

Cinnamon

If you struggle with maintaining a balance in your cholesterol level, then adding cinnamon to your juices will help you to reduce the level of LDL and prevent infections and diabetes from occurring in your body thanks to its blood sugar-regulating characteristics and anti-infectious compounds.

Cloves

These are packed with extremely high vitamin and mineral contents, as well as fibers, to help maintain the body's health and aid in digestion. As the body ages, it might get more prone to accumulating gasses and toxins; cloves help in a great deal promoting the expulsion of such problems.

Vanilla

Vanilla has been used for a long time for its mesmerizing scent, which surprisingly helps to encourage weight loss! Aside from being an effective weight loss agent, vanilla can also eliminate feelings of nausea, helping the whole body to relax and control symptoms of anxiety.

Nutmeg

Insomnia is an increasing problem that has been haunting the sleep of many, including you perhaps! The quality that puts nutmeg on this list is its ability to greatly aid in making you fall asleep and increase the potency of your immune system. If you are a beauty queen, then you should be happy to know that this also goes as far as to brighten your skin and complexion!

Black Pepper

A spice that was once used as a currency, black pepper has the characteristics of stimulating a very intense flavor on top of your tongue which encourages the release of hydrochloric acid, thereby enhancing your digestion capabilities while increasing protein and food absorption as well.

Tellicherry Peppercorn

If you want to add a soft aroma to your juices, then you can't go wrong with Tellicherry Peppercorn. You might've heard about these from multiple cooking shows, well, these were a major export for the British East India Company back in the days and are primarily famous for their hypnotic aroma.

Cumin

Hailing from the Mediterranean region, this spice is a great source of iron. But recent studies also concluded that this spice helps to lower the glucose level of blood and water down pains from arthritis joints.

Oregano

When you hear of oregano, you are reminded of Italian pizzas and Super Mario! But you can also put pinches of oregano in your juice to get the extra benefit of fending off bacteria by creating an invisible barrier against E. coli, listeria, and even salmonella. It has been proven that oregano oil is specifically the most effective antimicrobial agent available.

Storing Your Juices for Later Use

While storing juices is good, you should know that there are various juices with enzymes, carotene, chlorophyll, lipids, etc., that tend to have their nutrients evaporate minutes after they are turned into juices. So, while you can store juices for later use, you won't be able to get the full range of benefits that that particular juice has to offer. The length for which juice can be stored depends on a few striking factors, and the type of juicer that you use plays an important role here. When planning the storage of your juices, you should keep an eye out for juicers with the lowest RPM, as these help to minimally oxidize the juice as it is being produced, allowing it to be stored for longer later.

The best solution for storing your juices is to use glass containers that are generally designed with a wide mouth with a capacity of 16 or 32 ounces. Alternatively, you can also go for stainless steel water bottles. But keep in mind - refrain from using plastic, as they have the tendency to leach into the food that you are storing inside them and fill them up with toxins.

If you are thinking of storing your juices for even longer, you can go to another great length and freeze your juices in either ice trays or large milk jars. But this is not recommended as the juices will undergo even larger degradation in freezers.

Tips for Juicing Success

Read the Manual

I definitely recommend reading the manual of your juicer before you get started in order to fully understand how your juicer operates, as well as the purpose of each part.

Don't Overload the Juicer

Resist the urge to rush or overload the juicer. If you cram in too many pieces of produce or try and force the produce through too quickly, it can jam. Be patient and use small, thin pieces one at a time.

Make It Fit

Some juicers have a narrow juicing chute, so you'll want to make sure your produce is cut thinly enough to feed through the juicer. For greens, it's helpful to roll, fold, or bunch the greens before feeding them through.

Reuse the Pulp

It may feel like juicing is wasteful because you're left with an abundance of pulp. However, there are many fantastic ways to reuse the pulp, such as making recipes (check out the recipes in this book marked "Made with Juice Pulp") or using the pulp as compost to nourish your garden.

Aim for Green

If juicing for health is your goal, aim to make your juices mostly greens and herbs, with a small amount of fruit to sweeten them up. If you're watching your blood sugar levels, stick with lower-sugar fruits such as green apples, kiwis, or berries.

Rotate Ingredients

It's normal to find a favorite juice combination and want to stick with it. However, to ensure you provide your body with an array of nutrients, aim to try new ingredients. This will also provide a variety of flavors, so you don't get bored.

Choose Organic When Possible

Pesticides, herbicides, synthetic fertilizers, and chemicals can end up in your juice if you use conventional produce. When possible, choose organic produce to avoid these unwanted additives.

Adjust for Taste

If you're not enjoying the flavor of your juice, include one or two pieces of fruit, such as an apple or orange. Another thing to remember is that your palate and taste buds can change over time. What didn't taste good last year could become this year's favorite!

Cold Juice Tastes Best

Your juice will likely be at room temperature right after you've finished juicing. I like to put my juice in the refrigerator or freezer for about five minutes to quickly chill it, and then add it to a large glass with lots of ice. Crisp, cold juice tastes best! If you've been drinking room-temperature juice, try it chilled—you'll love how much more refreshing it tastes.

Freeze Fruits and Veggies

For blended juices, I recommend freezing produce. In addition to improving the texture of blended juices, freezing will help your fruits and veggies last longer, as well as free up space in your refrigerator. You can chop and freeze broccoli, zucchini, cauliflower, and even kale.

Chapter 2: Detoxing Recipes

Chard Lime Green Juice

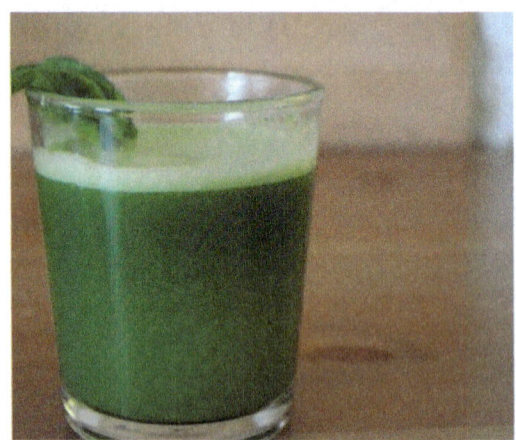

Preparation Time: 10 minutes

Servings: 4

Ingredients:

1 medium apple

1/2 lemon

2 medium cucumber

4 chard leaves

Directions:

Add all ingredients into the juicer and blend.

Serve and enjoy.

Arugula Orange Mint Juice

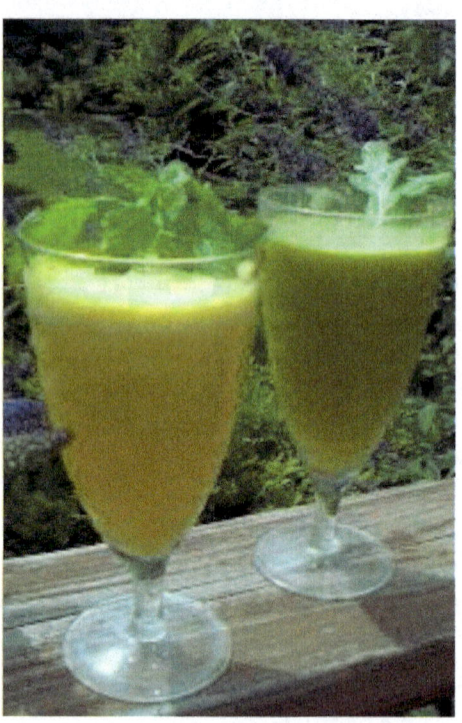

Preparation Time: 10 minutes

Servings: 2

Ingredients:

2 oranges

1/2 cucumber

1 handful mint

1 handful arugula

Directions:

Add all ingredients into the juicer and blend.

Serve and enjoy.

Tangy Beety Detox Juice

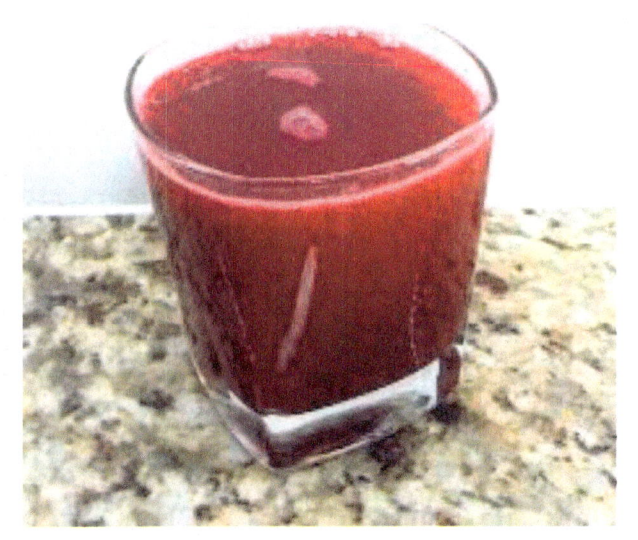

Preparation Time: 15 minutes

Servings: 2

Ingredients:

1 beetroot (chopped)

3 carrots (chopped)

2 leaves red cabbage

½ Lemon

1 orange – 1

¼ pineapple (chopped)

2 handfuls of spinach

Directions:

Push all the ingredients through the juicer and juice.

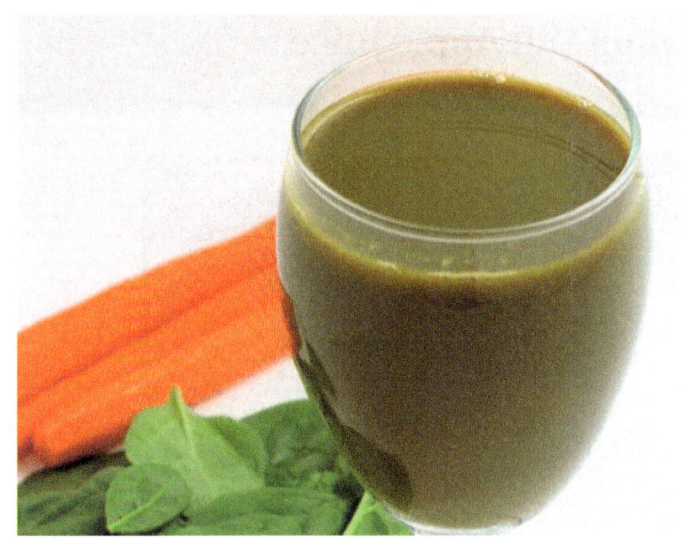

Spinach Orange Celery Juice

Preparation Time: 10 minutes

Servings: 2

Ingredients:

1 1/2 cups fresh spinach

1/2-inch fresh ginger

1 celery stalk

2 oranges, peeled

1 lime, peeled

2 lemons, peeled

1 green apple

Directions:

Add all ingredients into the juicer and blend.

Serve immediately and enjoy.

Fennel Dill Apple Juice

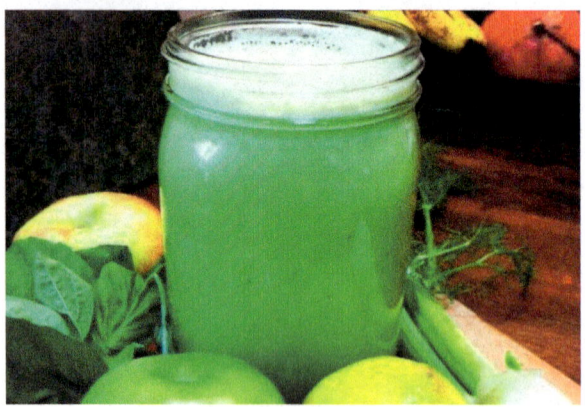

Preparation Time: 10 minutes

Servings: 2

Ingredients:

1/2 lemon, peeled

1 cucumber

2 green apples

4 tbsp fresh dill

1 cup baby spinach

2 fennel bulbs

Directions:

Add all ingredients into the juicer and blend.

Serve and enjoy.

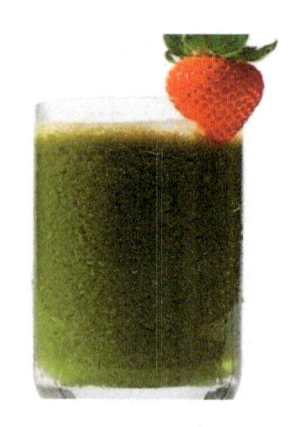

Servings: 2

Ingredients:

1 apple

Handful fresh parsley

Handful fresh spinach

10 strawberries

Directions:

Add all ingredients into the juicer and blend.

Serve and enjoy.

Apple Strawberry Spinach Juice

Preparation Time: 10 minutes

Green Detox Juice

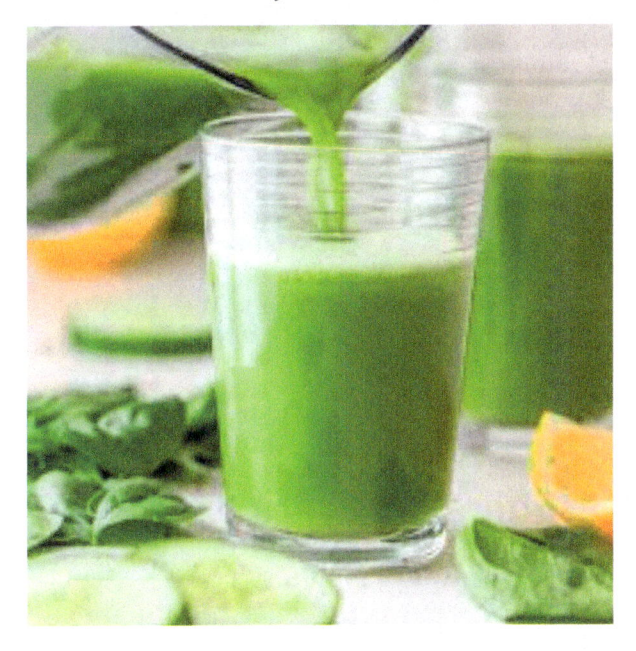

Preparation Time: 15 minutes

Servings: 4

Ingredients:

5 small carrots, chopped
1/2 cup wheatgrass
1 sprig parsley
2 sticks of celery
1/2 beet, with top
1 large apple, chopped

Directions:

Push the parsley and wheatgrass through the juicer alternating with the carrot. Now alternate the apple, celery, and beet. This is a nutrient-dense drink packed full of healthy chlorophyll and antioxidants. Wheatgrass is high in Indole which helps prevent cancer. It is high in many beneficial enzymes.

Fresh Cilantro Lettuce Orange juice

Preparation Time: 10 minutes

Servings: 2

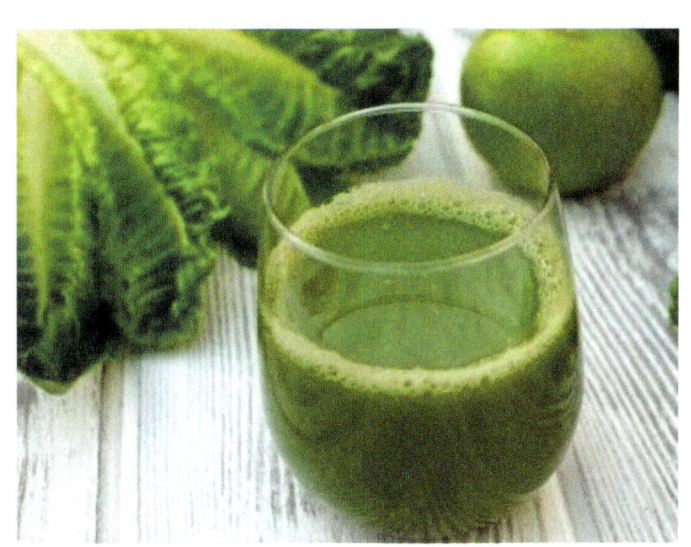

Ingredients:

2 oranges

1 handful fresh cilantro

1 head romaine lettuce

2 kale leaves

2 celery stalks

Directions:

Add all ingredients into the juicer and blend.

Serve and enjoy.

Coconut Pineapple Lettuce Juice

Preparation Time: 10 minutes

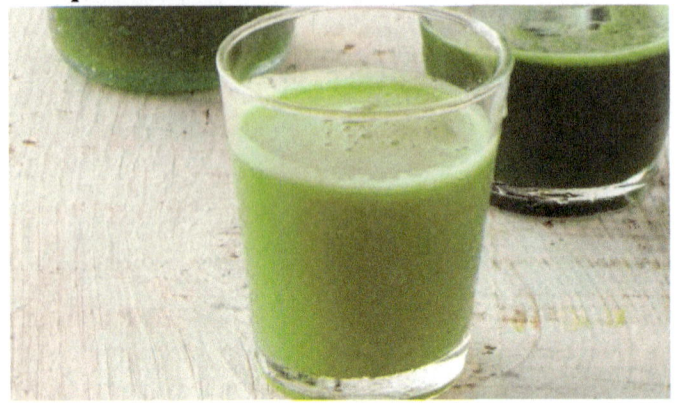

Servings: 2

Ingredients:

1/4 cup coconut water

1/2-inch fresh ginger

2 cups pineapple

2 celery stalks

1 heart of romaine lettuce

1/2 cucumber

Directions:

Add all ingredients into the juicer and blend.

Serve and enjoy.

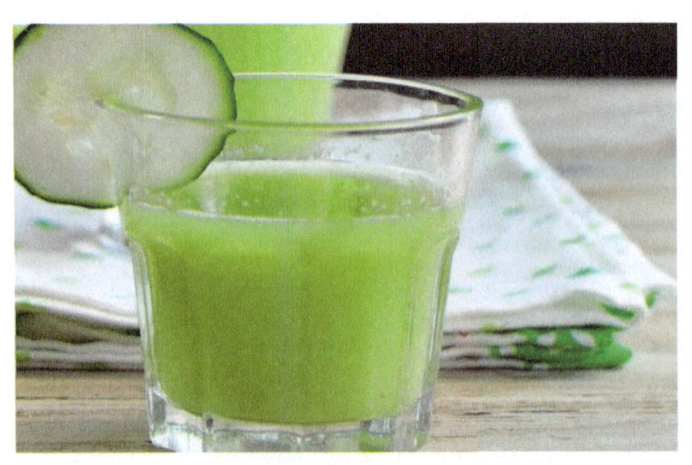

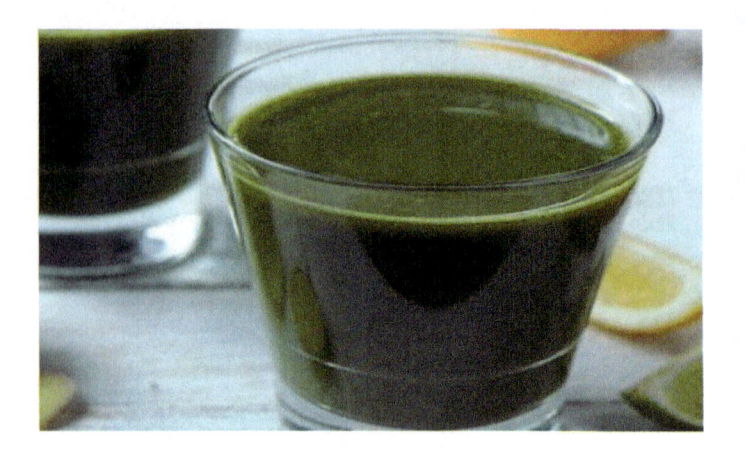

Refreshing Lean Green Juice

Preparation Time: 10 minutes

Servings: 5

Ingredients:

10 mint leaves

1 cup fresh spinach

1 fresh lime juice

1/2 pear

1/2 cucumber

1/2 cup pineapple

Ice cubes

1 tsp honey

Directions:

Add all ingredients into the juicer and blend.

Serve and enjoy.

Pear Lemon Cucumber Juice

Preparation Time: 10 minutes

Servings: 2

Ingredients:

1 cucumber

1/2 lemon

2 medium pears

2 lettuce heads

Directions:

Add all ingredients into the juicer and blend.

Serve immediately and enjoy.

Fruity Spinach Detox Juice

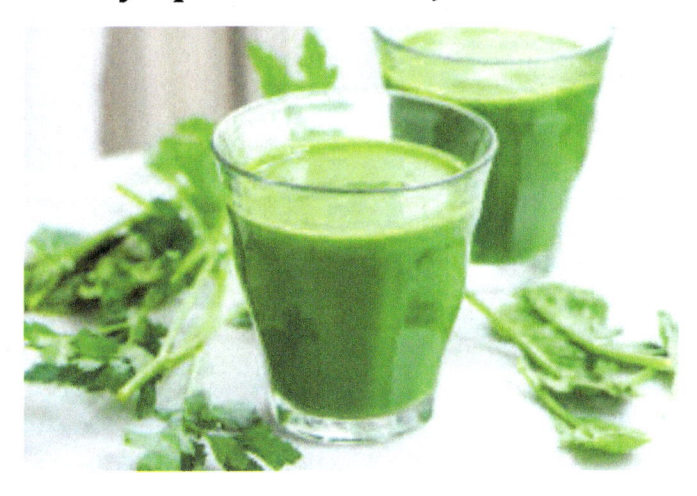

Preparation Time: 10 minutes

Servings: 2

Ingredients:

3 Packham pears (chopped)

3 Granny Smith apples (chopped)

3.5oz baby spinach

5 fresh mint sprigs

Directions:

Push all the ingredients through the juicer and juice it.

Harmless Purple Passion Juice

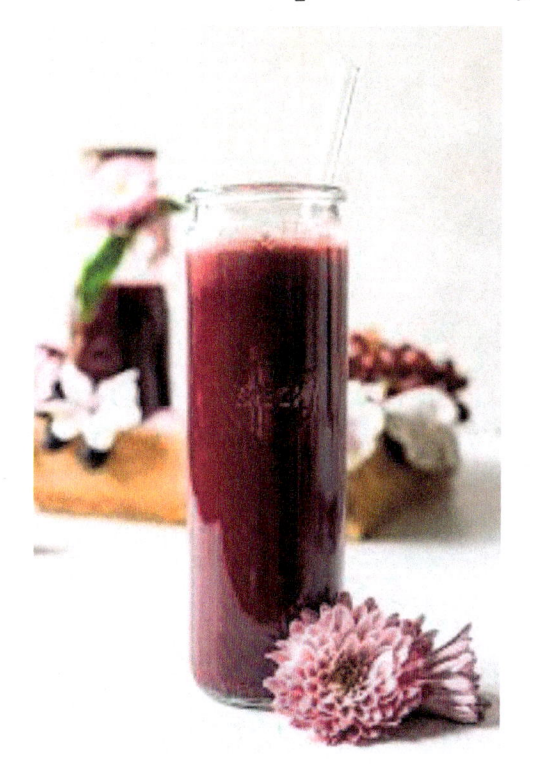

Preparation Time: 10 minutes

Servings: 2

Ingredients:

4 medium-sized apples

¼ head of small red cabbage

1 whole lime fruit

Directions:

Add the ingredients to your juicer or centrifuge.

Process them thoroughly until you have a smooth juice.

Pour the drink into a glass and give it a nice shake. Chill and serve!

Dreamy Watermelon Juice

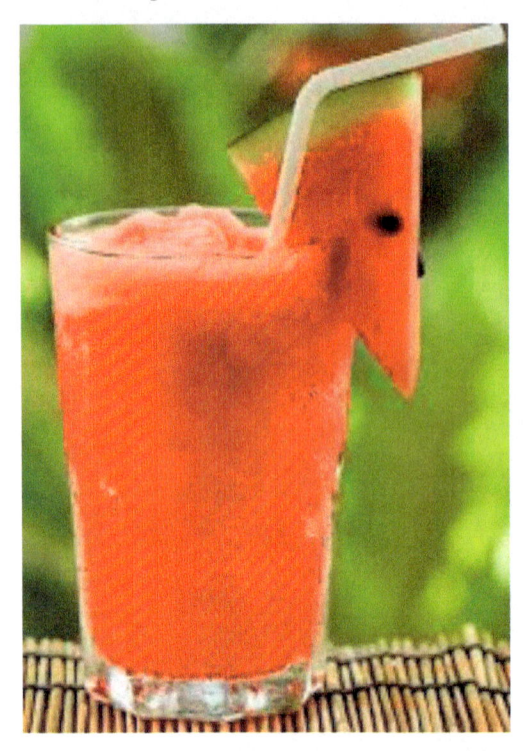

Preparation Time: 20 minutes

Servings: 2

Ingredients:

½ of a lime fruit

1 medium-sized peach

7 peppermint leaves

1 whole cup of strawberry

2 cups of diced watermelon

Directions:

Add the ingredients to your juicer or centrifuge. Process them thoroughly until you have a smooth juice.

Pour the drink into a glass and give it a nice shake. Chill and serve!

Liver Cleanse Juice

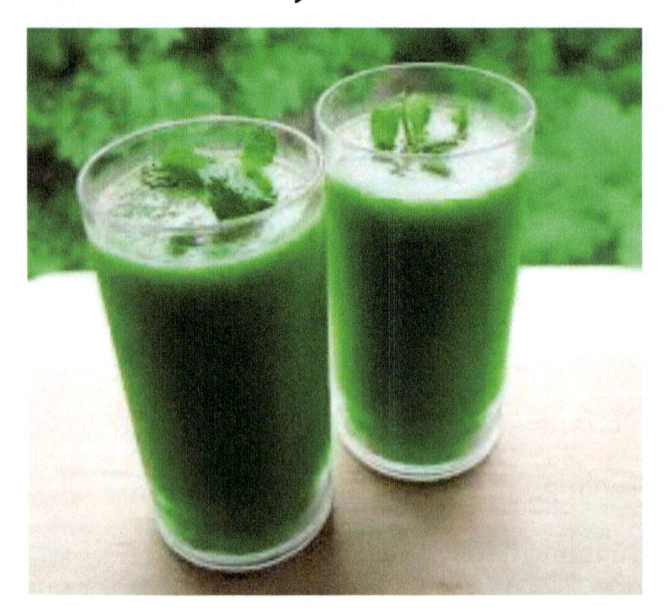

Preparation Time: 10 minutes

Servings: 3

Ingredients:

½ red cabbage

1 carrot

1 celery stalk

1 apple

1-inch fresh ginger root

A handful parsley

A handful dandelion

Directions:

Put all of the ingredients into a blender and pulse for 2 minutes until it's a smooth texture.

Serve chilled.

The Secret Pink Juice

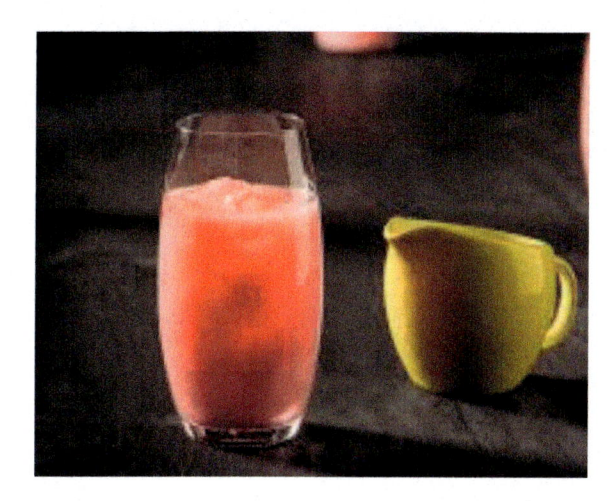

Preparation Time: 10 minutes

Servings: 5

Ingredients:

1 medium-sized apple

1 orange fruit

1 whole cup of strawberry

1 whole cup of diced watermelon

Directions:

Add the ingredients to your juicer or centrifuge.

Process them thoroughly until you have a smooth juice.

Pour the drink into a glass and give it a nice shake.

Chill and serve!

Green Goddess Detox Juice

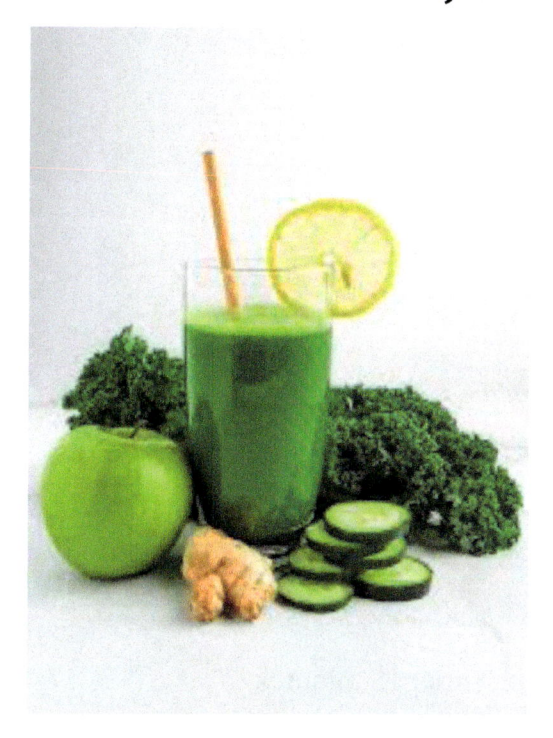

Preparation Time: 10 minutes

Servings: 2

Ingredients:

10 spinach leaves

½ cup parsley

1 celery stalk

½ cucumber

Directions:

Push all the ingredients through the juicer and juice.

Chill.

Golden Detox Juice

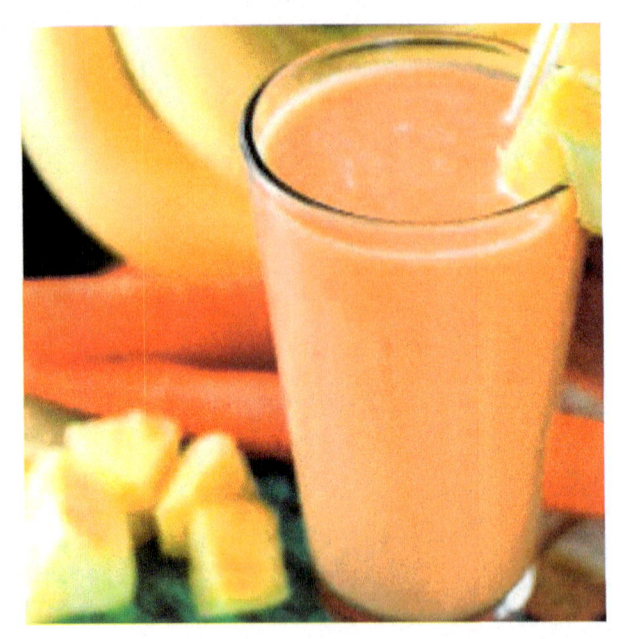

Preparation Time: 15 minutes

Servings: 4

Ingredients:

1 golden beetroot (chopped)

3 carrots (chopped)

4 celery stalks

½ cucumber

1 ginger root (1" piece)

1 bosc pear (chopped)

Directions:

Push all the ingredients through the juicer and juice.

Sweet Beet Detox Juice

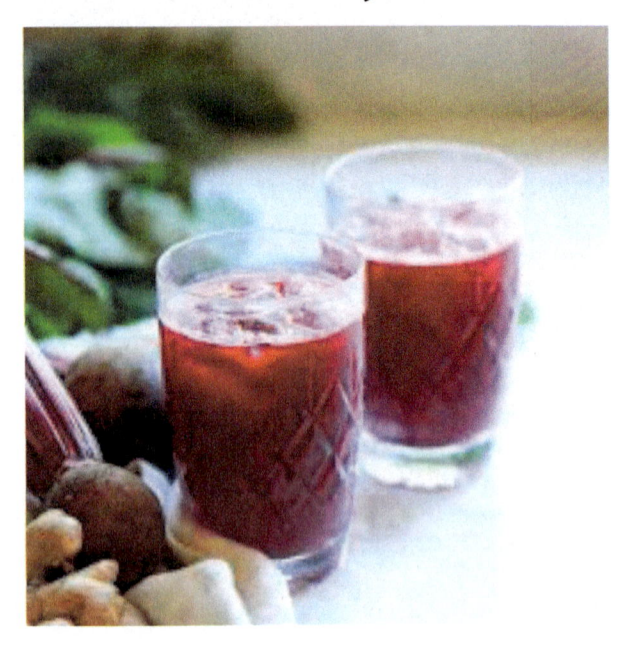

Preparation Time: 15 minutes

Servings: 4

Ingredients:

2 apples (chopped)

4 carrots (chopped)

1 beetroot

3 celery stalks

½ cucumber

1 Ginger root (1" piece)

Directions:

Push all the ingredients through the juicer and juice.

Super Detox Juice

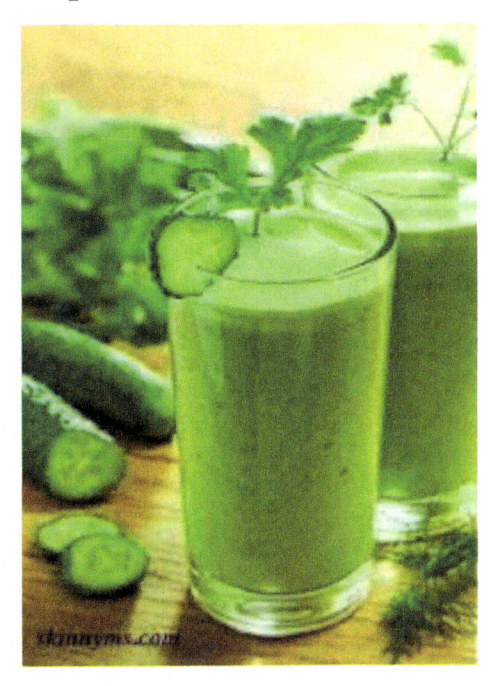

Preparation Time: 10 minutes

Servings: 3

Ingredients:

½ cabbage

4 celery stalks

4 carrots

½ cilantro bunch

1 beet with greens

1 fennel bulb

1 raw ginger

1 whole lemon

Directions:

Put all of the ingredients into a blender and pulse for 2 minutes until it's a smooth texture. Serve chilled.

Citrus Beet Detox Juice

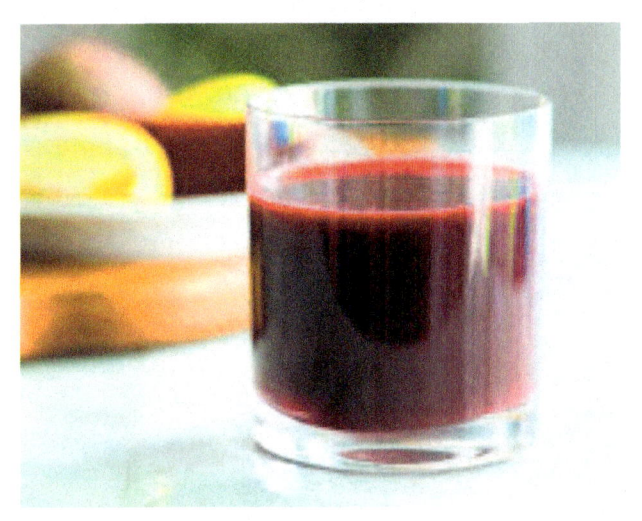

Preparation Time: 15 minutes

Servings: 4

Ingredients:

2 apples (chopped)

2 carrots (chopped)

1 beetroot (chopped)

1 celery stalks

2 peeled oranges

1 ginger slice (1" piece)

Directions:

Chill all the ingredients.

Push all the ingredients through the juicer and juice.

Serve over crushed ice.

The Root Detox Juice

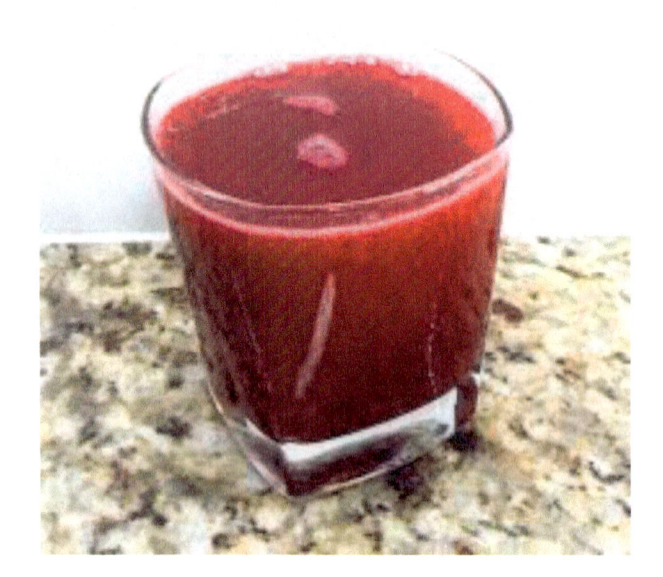

Preparation Time: 15 minutes

Servings: 4

Ingredients:

10 carrots (chopped)

1 beetroot (chopped)

1 sweet Potato (chopped)

Directions:

Push all the ingredients through the juicer first the beet, then sweet potato, and then the carrots.

Juice it!

Chapter 3 : Juices for Ailments

Fennel Fabulous Juice

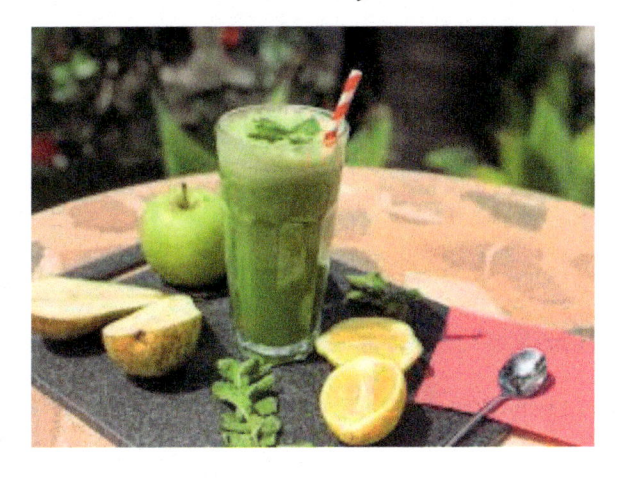

Preparation Time: 10 minutes

Servings: 3

Ingredients:

1 fennel bulb

2 handfuls of Swiss chard

1 celery stalk

2 granny smith apples

2 kiwis

1 pear

½ inch of ginger

Directions:

Put all of the ingredients into a blender and pulse for 2 minutes until it's a smooth texture. Serve chilled.

The Green Man Juice

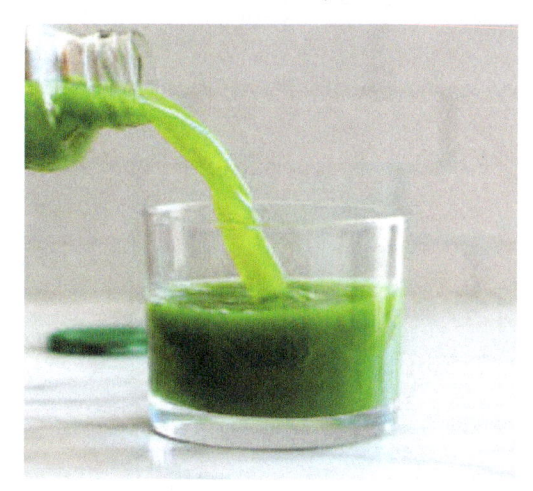

Preparation Time: 10 minutes

Servings: 3

Ingredients:

½ bunch of kale

4 stalks of celery

3 small chunks of radish

½ bunch of cabbage

1 cucumber

4 sprigs of cilantro

½ lemon

Directions:

Put all of the ingredients into a blender and pulse for 2 minutes until it's a smooth texture. Serve chilled.

Sunset Juice

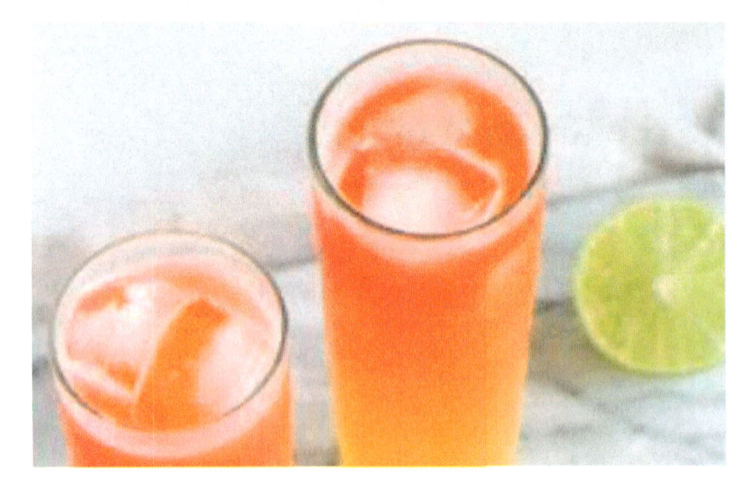

Preparation Time: 10 minutes

Servings: 4

Ingredients

1 large carrot

1 medium orange, with rind

1 5-inch sweet potato

2 medium apples

2 medium beetroots

1 medium red bell pepper

Directions:

Extract the juices from all the ingredients and mix together. Place in a glass and enjoy.

Parsnip Juice

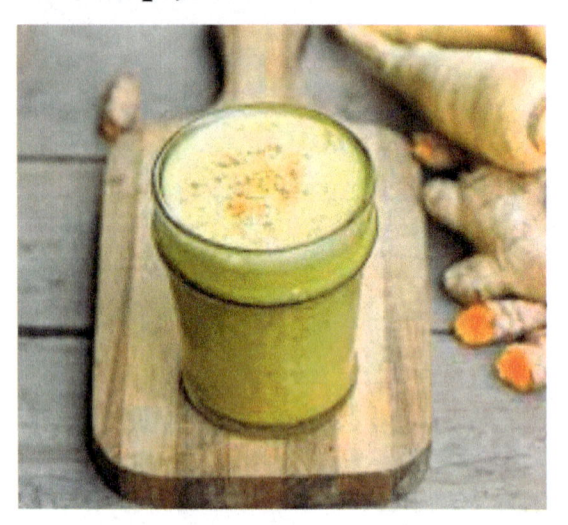

Preparation Time: 10 minutes

Servings: 4

Ingredients:

2 large parsnips

2 sweet potatoes

1 cup pineapple, peeled

1 mandarin orange, peeled

1 1-inch ginger

Directions:

Press all the ingredients through a juicer. Mix the juices together before serving.

Kale-Cium Juice

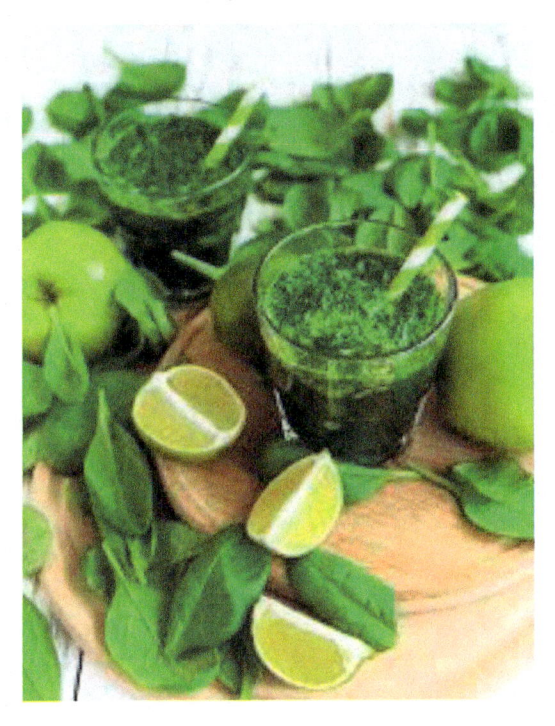

Preparation Time: 15 minutes

Servings: 4

Ingredients:

1 apple (chopped)

1 red bell pepper

4 kale leaves

1 cup collard greens

1 fresh cilantro

3 handful carrots (chopped)

Directions:

Push all the ingredients through the juicer and juice.

Blood-Building Elixir Juice

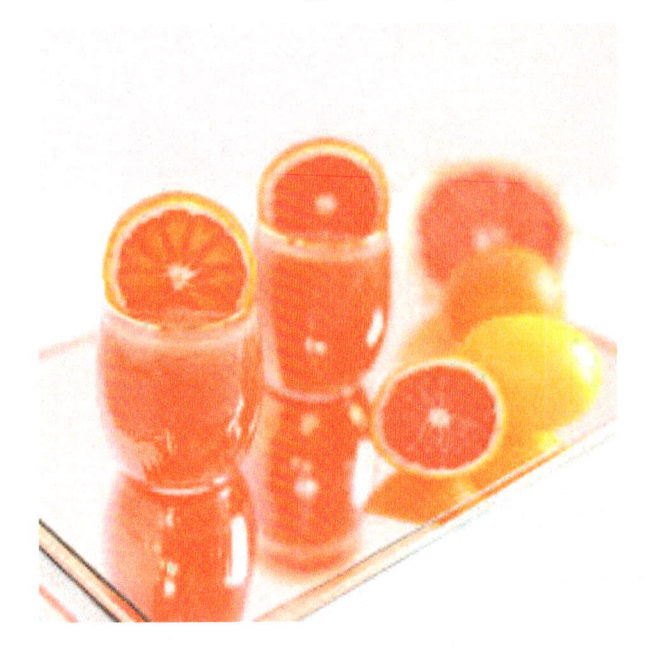

Preparation Time: 10 minutes

Servings: 3

Ingredients

15 leaf of beet greens

1 beetroot beet of 3-inch diameter

7 medium-sized carrots

2 leaf of kale measuring 8-12-inches

Directions:

Add the ingredients to your juicer or centrifuge.

Process them thoroughly until you have a smooth juice.

Pour the drink into a glass and give it a nice shake.

Chill and serve!

Colon Friendly Green Juice

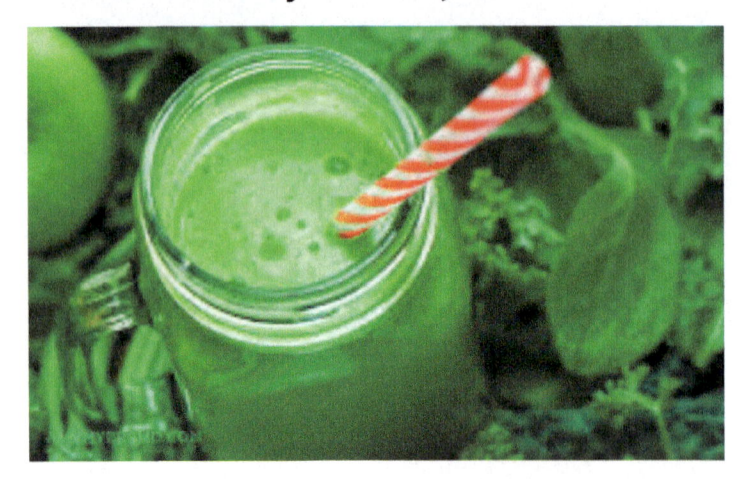

Preparation Time: 10 minutes

Servings: 2

Ingredients:

3 medium-sized apples

4 large celery stalks

¼ A thumb of ginger root

½ a fruit of lemon with rinds included

1 large, peeled orange

5 handfuls of spinach

Directions:

Peel the skin of your orange if you want to avoid a bitter flavor.

Add the ingredients to your juicer or centrifuge.

Process them thoroughly until you have a smooth juice.

Pour the drink into a glass and give it a nice shake.

Chill and serve!

Intestine Scrubbing Pomegranate Green Juice

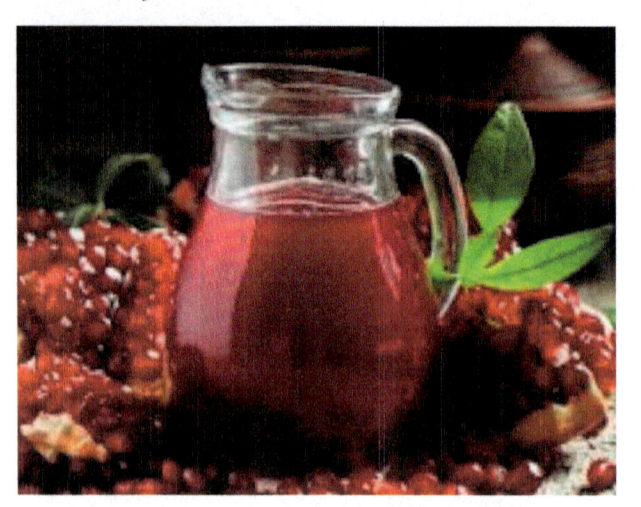

Preparation Time: 10 minutes

Servings: 2

Ingredients

1 medium-sized apple

4 medium-sized celery stalks

½ of a cucumber

2 cups of grapes

1 cup of pomegranate

4 cups of spinach

Directions:

Add the ingredients to your juicer or centrifuge.

Process them thoroughly until you have a smooth juice.

Pour the drink into a glass and give it a nice shake.

Chill and serve!

Minty Orange Juice

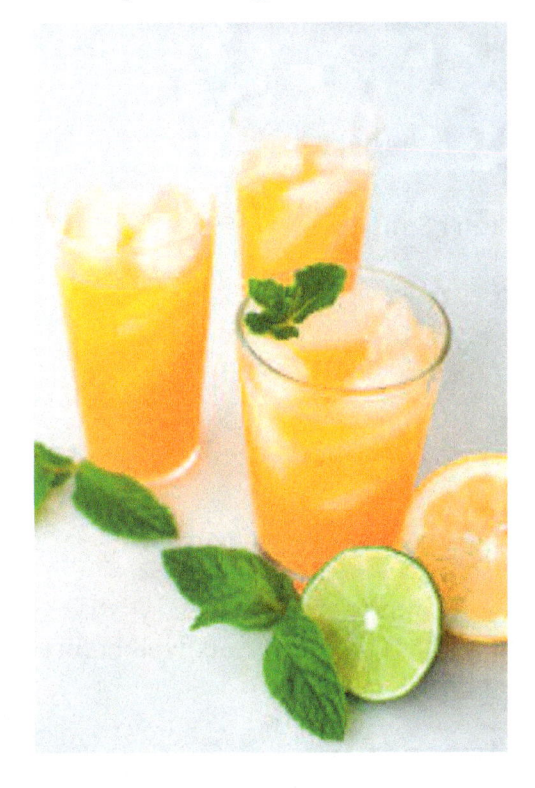

Preparation Time: 15 minutes

Servings: 4

Ingredients:

¼ teaspoon ground cinnamon

½ cup coconut water

1 fennel bulb

1 lemon

1 oranges (peeled)

2 pears

10 peppermint leaves

Directions:

Push all the ingredients through the juicer and juice.

Creamsicle Juice

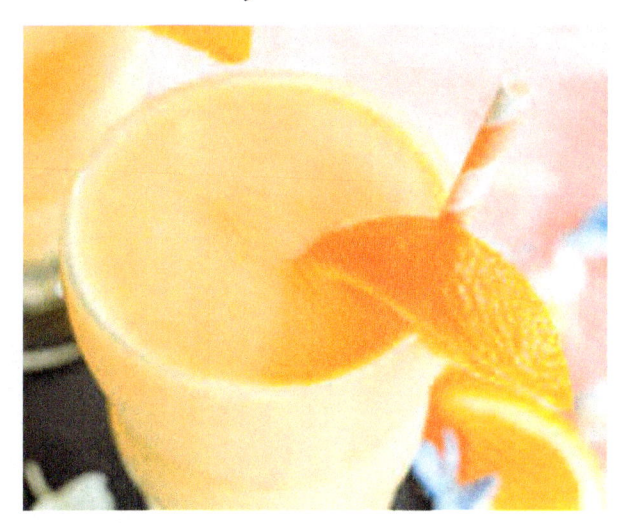

Preparation Time: 15 minutes

Servings: 4

Ingredients:

2 apples

3 celery stalks

1 orange (peeled)

2 pears

1 sweet potato

Directions:

Push all the ingredients through the juicer and juice.

Very Berry Juice

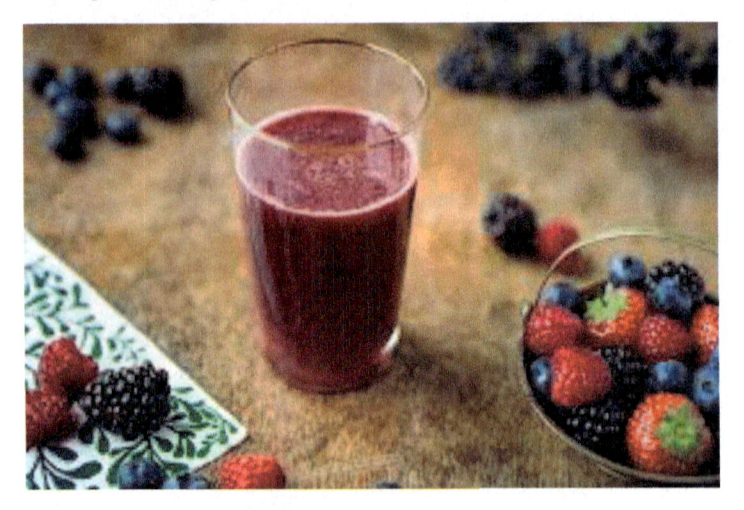

Preparation Time: 15 minutes

Servings: 4

Ingredients:

3 cups whole strawberries

2 large Granny Smith apples

½ lime, fruit only

Directions:

Place the strawberries, apples, and lime in a juicer. Place in a glass then serve.

Beet and Veggies Juice

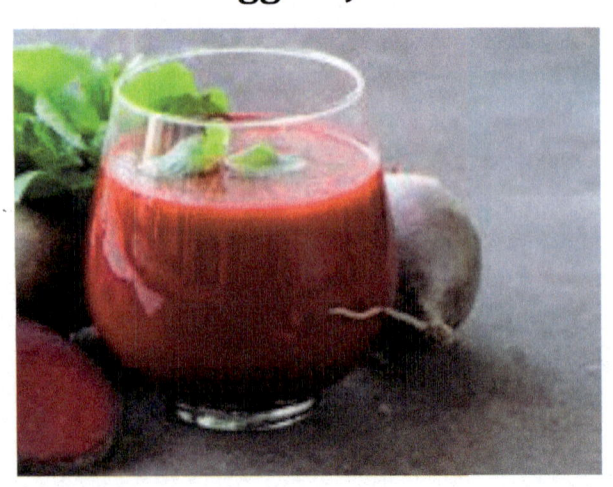

Preparation Time: 10 minutes

Servings: 4

Ingredients:

1 beetroot

1 large red Granny Smith apple

4 large carrots

3 large celery stalks

½ cucumber

1 ½-inch ginger

Directions:

Process the beet, apple, carrots, celery stalks, cucumber, and ginger in a juicer. Mix well before drinking.

Green Goddess Juice

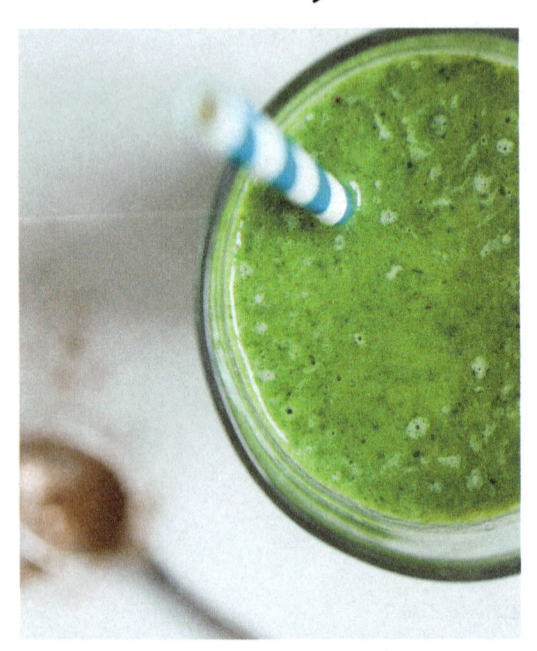

Preparation Time: 10 minutes

Servings: 3

Ingredients:

2 Granny Smith apples

1 bundle of spinach

2 celery stalks

1 cucumber

½ a lemon

1 inch of ginger

¼ of a pineapple skinned

Directions:

Put all of the ingredients into a blender and pulse for 2 minutes until it's a smooth texture.

Serve chilled.

Cucumber and Kale Lemonade Juice

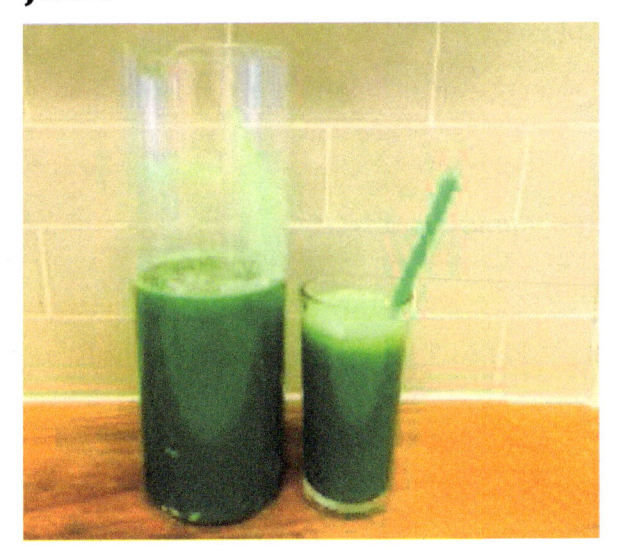

Preparation Time: 10 minutes

Servings: 4

Ingredients:

1 large cucumber

5 leaves of kale

2 medium apples

1 cup of spinach

1 lemon without the rind

Directions:

Place all of the ingredients in a juicer and mix well.

Jump Starter Juice

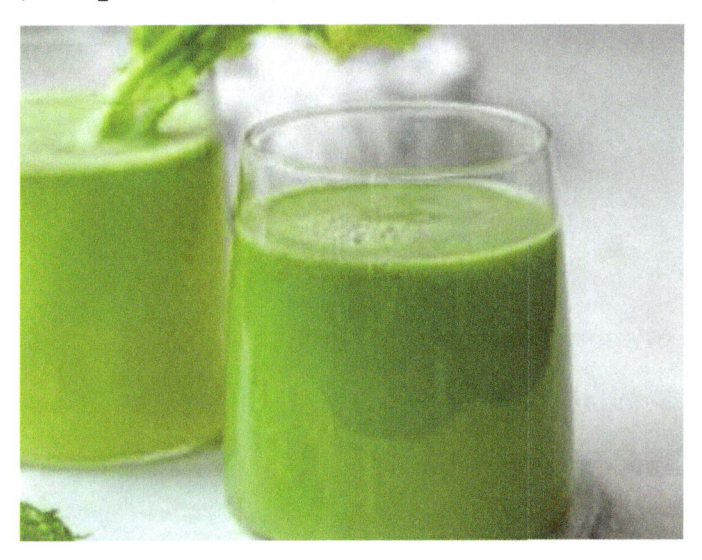

Preparation Time: 10 minutes

Servings: 3

Ingredients:

1 sweet potato

½ a beet with greens

2 carrots

2 stalks of celery

1 cucumber

2 apples

1 clove of garlic

Directions:

Put all of the ingredients into a blender and pulse for 2 minutes until it's a smooth texture. Serve chilled.

The Red Eye Juice

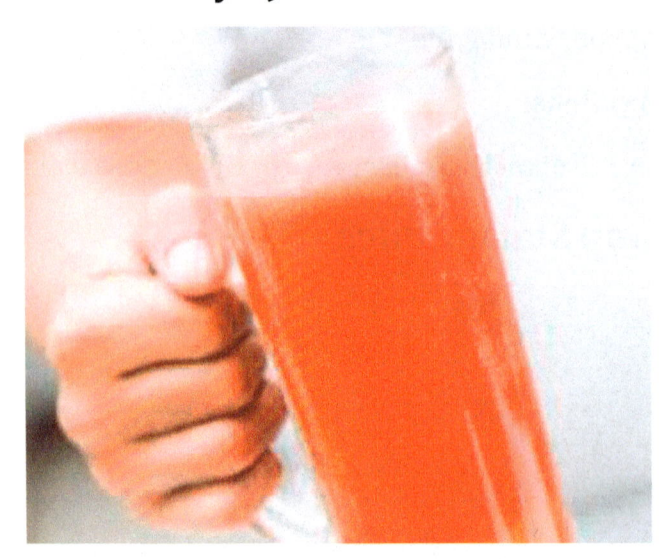

Preparation Time: 10 minutes

Servings: 3

Ingredients:

½ a red cabbage

1 beet with greens

½ sweet red pepper

3 carrots

1 apple

½ inch of ginger

Directions:

Put all of the ingredients into a blender and pulse for 2 minutes until it's a smooth texture. Serve chilled.

Hearty Spinach Juice

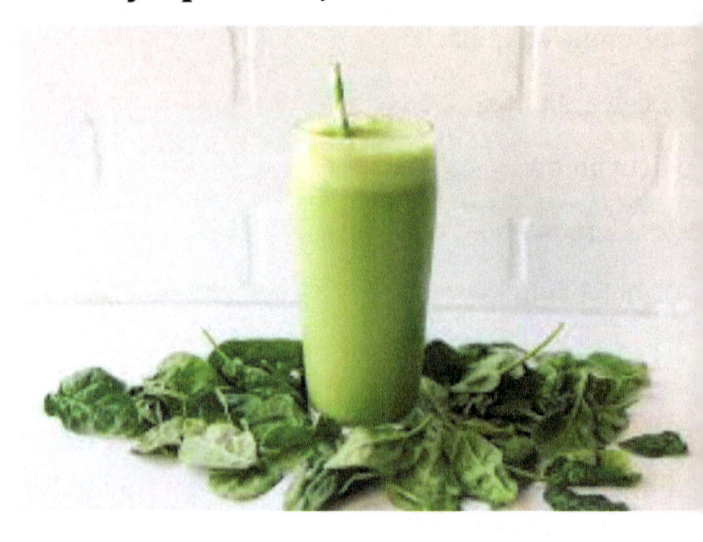

Preparation Time: 10 minutes

Servings: 4

Ingredients:

1 cup spinach

2 leaves of kale

1 handful of parsley

2 medium apples

Directions:

Juice the greens with the apples and mix well.

The Oprah Green Juice

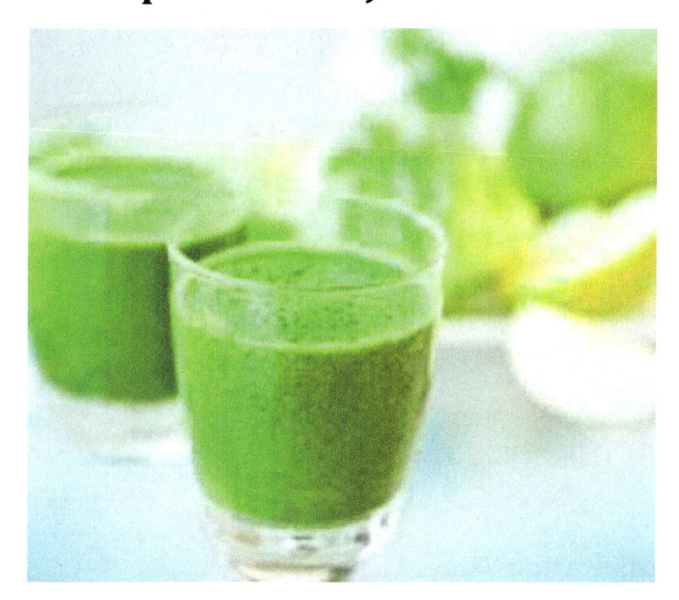

Preparation Time: 10 minutes

Servings: 4

Ingredients:

2 cups spinach

1 handful of parsley

3 stalks of celery

1 medium cucumber

1 whole lime

½ lemon fruit

2 medium apples

1 1-inch ginger

Directions:

Put the spinach, parsley, celery, cucumber, lime, lemon, apples, and ginger through a juicer. For a sweeter flavor, you may include extra apples. Mix then serve immediately.

Ginger and Lemon Juice

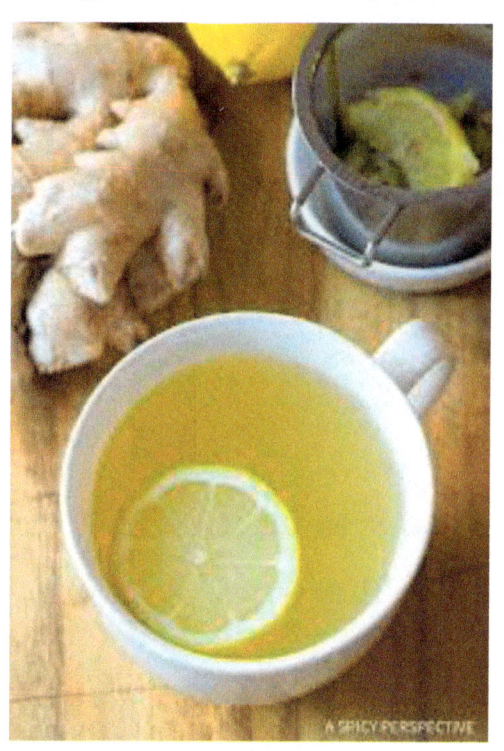

Preparation Time: 10 minutes

Servings: 4

Ingredients:

1 1-inch ginger

1 lemon

2 medium carrots

2 medium apples

Directions:

Juice all the ingredients together. Place in a glass and enjoy.

Mixed Carrot Juice

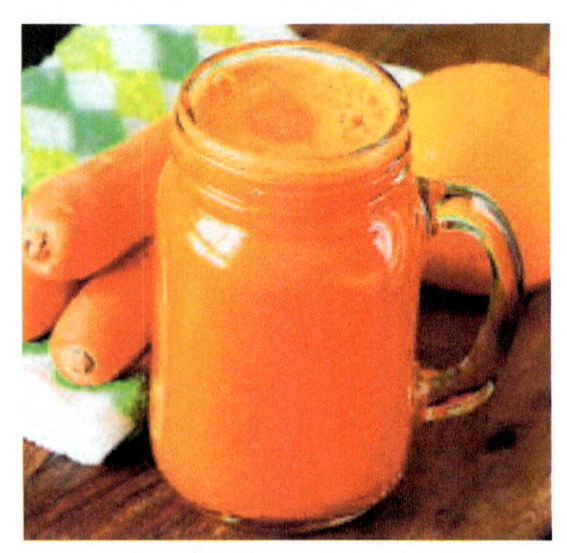

Preparation Time: 10 minutes

Servings: 4

Ingredients:

15 medium carrots

2 medium apples

2 small oranges

Directions:

Place the carrots in a juicer followed by the apples and oranges. Stir them together.

Alzheimer's Cure juice

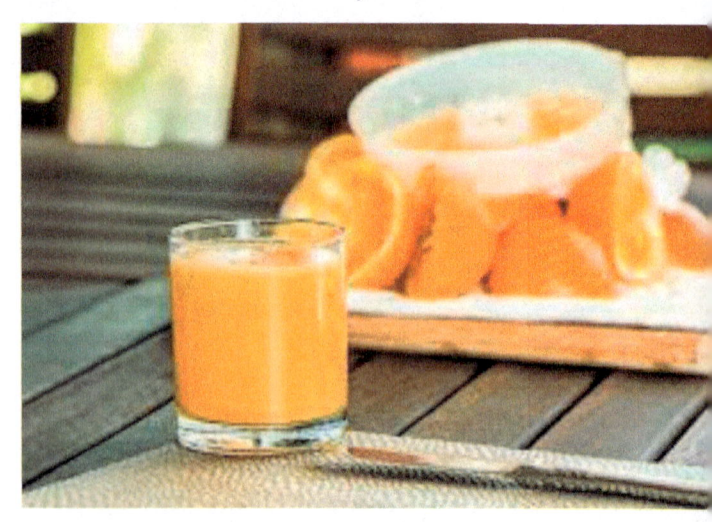

Preparation Time: 15 minutes

Servings: 4

Ingredients

2 large Granny Smith apples

8 large celery stalks

1 peeled lemon fruit

1 peeled orange fruit

Directions:

Add the ingredients to your juicer or centrifuge.

Process them thoroughly until you have a smooth juice.

Pour the drink into a glass and give it a nice shake.

Chill and serve!

Sweetened Broccoli Juice

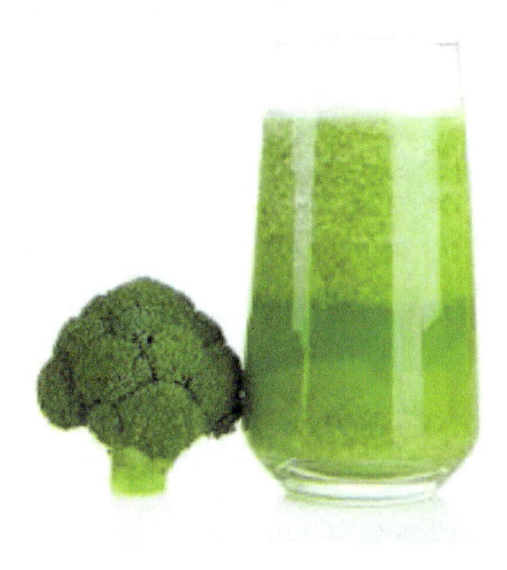

Preparation Time: 10 minutes

Servings: 4

Ingredients:

1 stalk broccoli

4 medium carrots

3 medium apples

Directions:

Juice the broccoli, carrots, and apples together. Shake then serve.

Avocado Green Juice

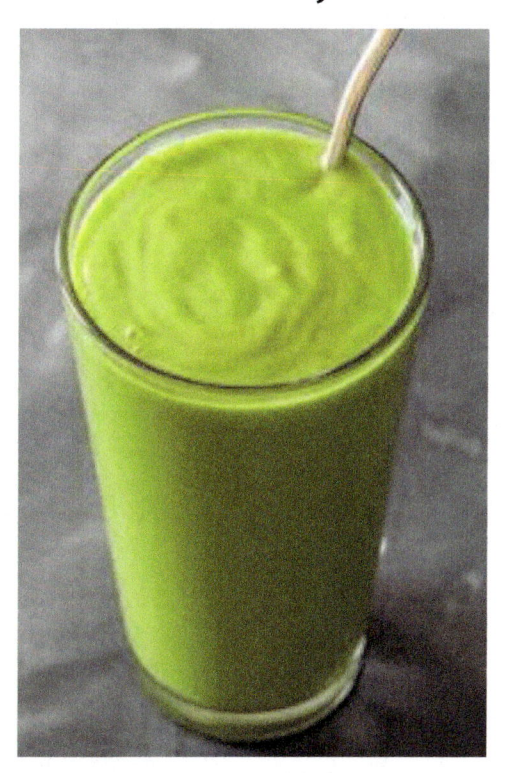

Preparation Time: 10 minutes

Servings: 4

Ingredients:

1 avocado, peeled and pitted

2 medium apples

12 grapes

3 large celery stalks

2 cups spinach

1 lime

Directions:

Place the ingredients in a centrifuge juicer until all the juices are blended in. You may drink this avocado blend to replace your lunch meal.

Bright Turmeric Juice

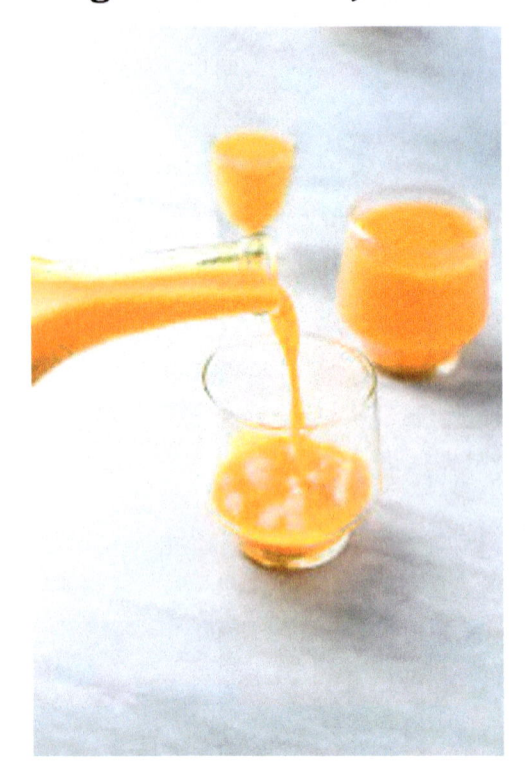

Preparation Time: 10 minutes

Servings: 4

Ingredients:

2 apples

3 celery stalks

3 carrots

1 ginger root (1" piece)

2 lemons (peeled)

2 pears

6 turmeric roots (1" pieces)

Directions:

Push all the ingredients through the juicer and juice.

Coconut Splash Juice

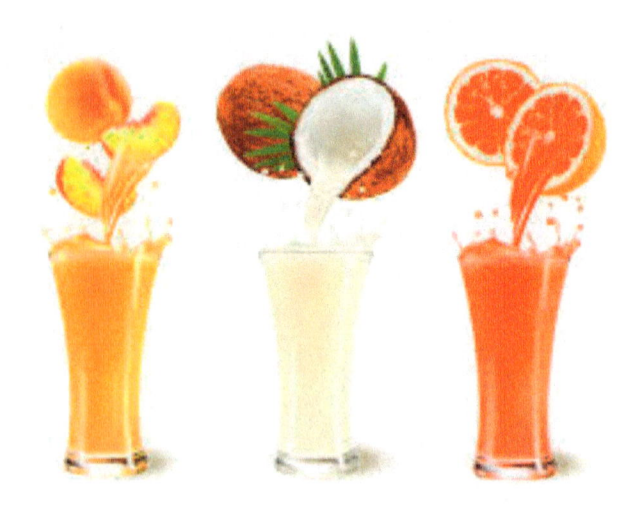

Preparation Time: 15 minutes

Servings: 4

Ingredients:

1 coconut kernel

2 oranges (peeled)

2 peaches

Directions:

Push all the ingredients through the juicer and juice.

Anti-Diabetic Greens Pear Smoothie

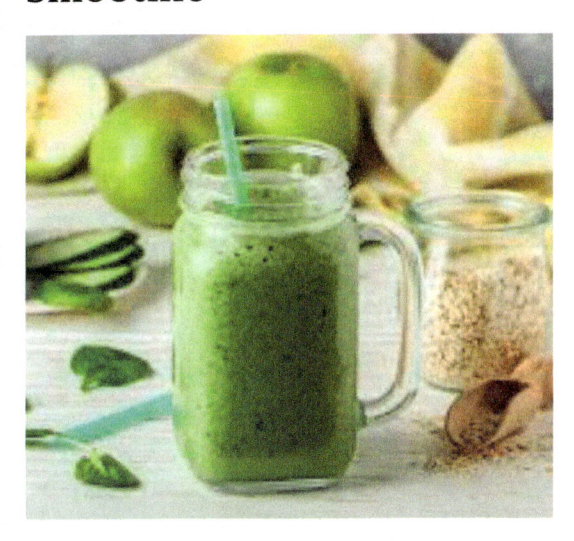

Preparation Time: 10 minutes

Servings: 4

Ingredients:

1 cupful of mesclun greens

1 cupful of almond milk

1 banana

1 pear

1 apple (cored)

1 teaspoonful of cinnamon

Directions:

Put leafy greens and water in a pitcher and blend until the mix becomes a consistent green.

Discontinue blending and put in residual ingredients. Turn on again and blend till it purees.

Dragon Fruit Juice

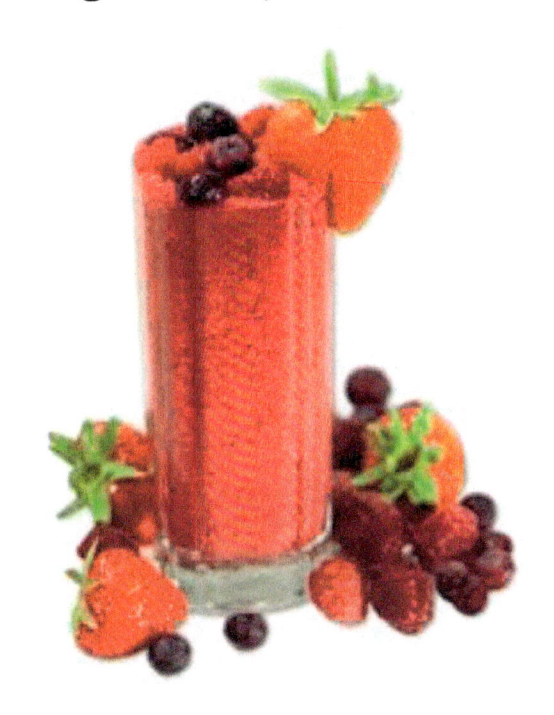

Preparation Time: 15 minutes

Servings: 4

Ingredients:

1 cup spinach

½ cup pitaya

1 banana

½ cup raspberries

1 date

1 ½ cup unsweetened almond milk

Cinnamon – Just a dash

Directions:

Add all the ingredients through the juicer and juice.

The Immune Juice

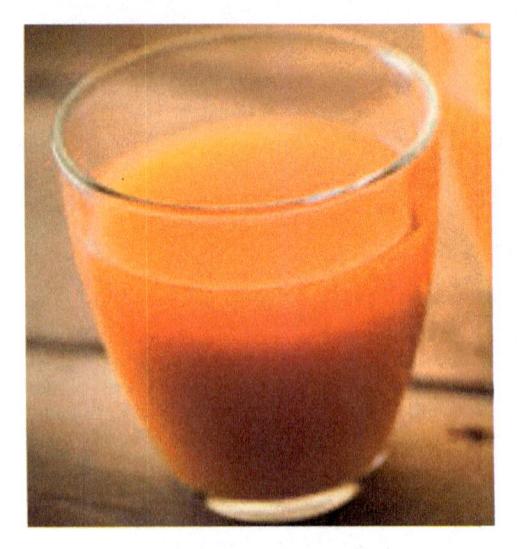

Preparation Time: 10 minutes

Servings: 3

Ingredients:

2 apple (chopped)

14 carrots (chopped)

2 orange (peeled)

Directions:

Push all the ingredients through the juicer and juice.

Golden Beet Juice

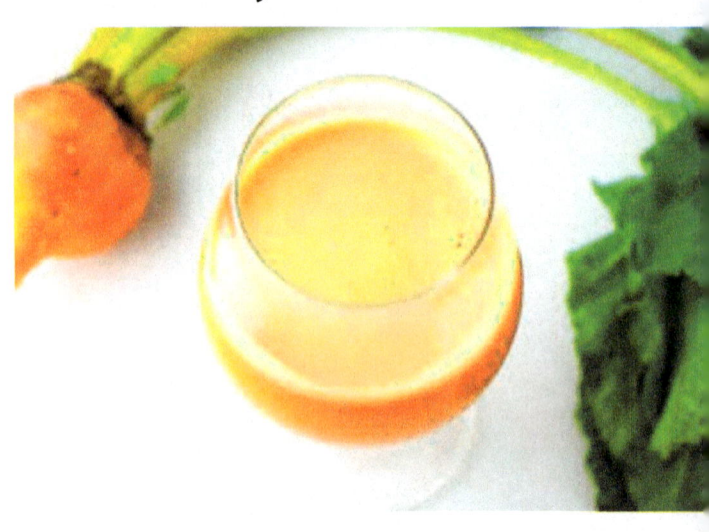

Preparation Time: 10 minutes

Servings: 3

Ingredients:

1 golden beet

3-carrots

4 celery stalks

½ cucumber

1 pear

1 ginger (1/2" piece)

Directions:

Push all the ingredients through the juicer and juice.

Red Peppered Juice

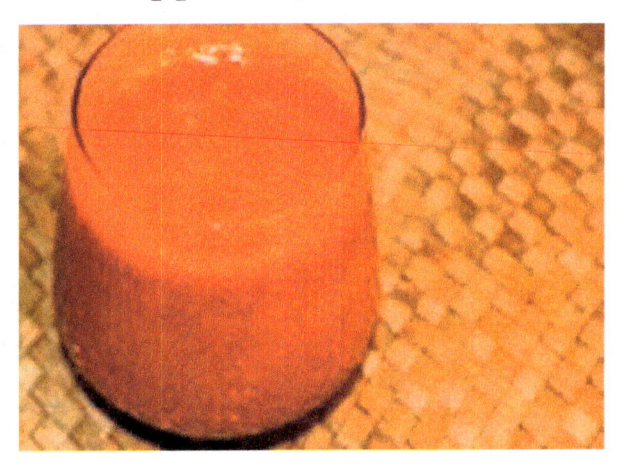

Preparation Time: 10 minutes

Servings: 3

Ingredients:

1 red bell pepper

1 cucumber

1 stalk of broccoli

1 carrot

2 stalks of celery

½ cup of jicama with skin

½ a lime with rind

1 beetroot

A handful of basil

1 jalapeño

1 tablespoon of chia seeds

Directions:

Put all of the ingredients into a blender and pulse for 2 minutes until it's a smooth texture. Serve chilled.

Apple and Celery Juice

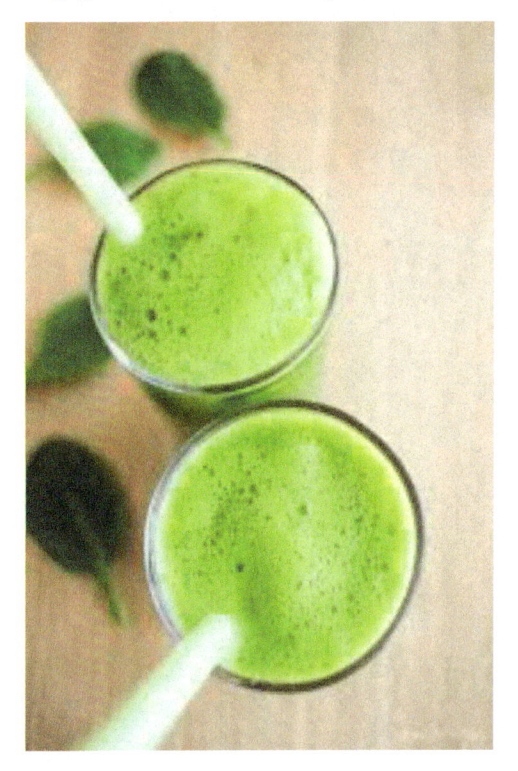

Preparation Time: 10 minutes

Servings: 4

Ingredients:

2 medium-sized Granny Smith apples

3 large celery stalks

Directions:

Process the apples and celery stalks in a juicer and mix well.

Sweet Beet Juice

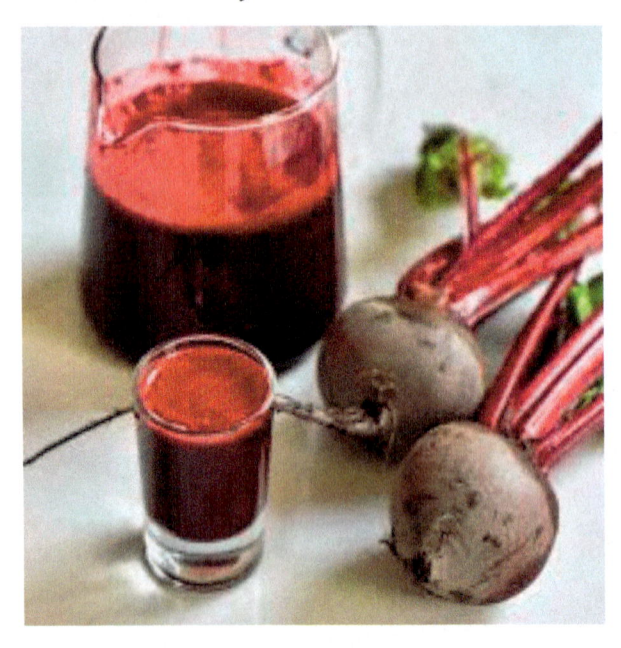

Preparation Time: 10 minutes

Servings: 4

Ingredients:

1 medium beetroot

1 5-inch sweet potato, peeled

2 medium apples

Directions:

Place the beetroot, sweet potato, and apples in a juicer. Stir together and place in a glass.

Cashew and Strawberry Juice

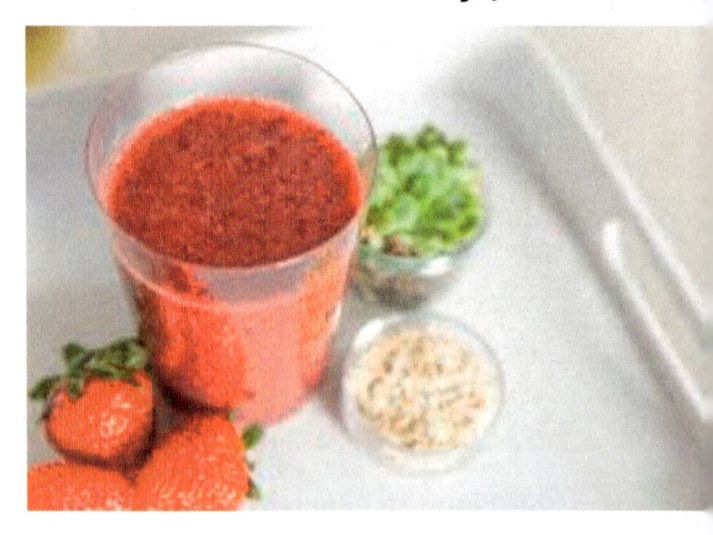

Preparation Time: 10 minutes

Servings: 3

Ingredients:

½ bananas

1 cup strawberries

¼ cup cashews

¼ cup coconut flakes

3 leaves mint

1 1/2 cups almond milk

Directions:

Add all the ingredients through the juicer and juice.

Peachy Immunity Juice

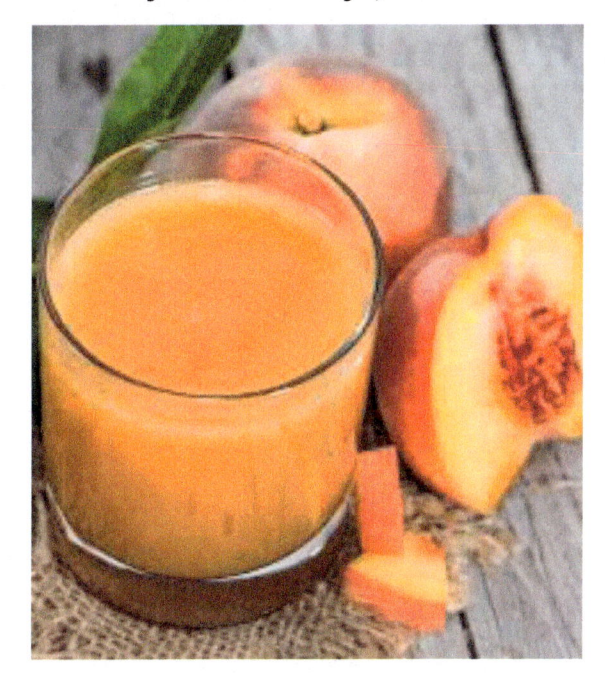

Preparation Time: 10 minutes

Servings: 3

Ingredients:

3 fresh basil leaves

14 carrots

½ lemon

5 peaches

Directions:

Add all the ingredients through the juicer in the order: basil, lemon, then peaches, and finally the carrots.

Juice it.

Chapter 4: Overall Health and Wellness Recipes

Magic Lemony Apple Juice

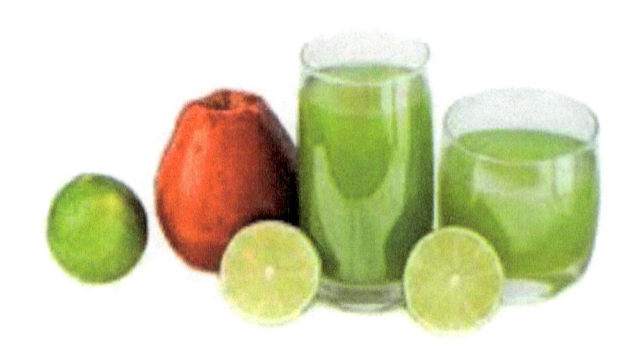

Preparation Time: 10 minutes

Servings: 3

Ingredients:

3 cups apple (cubed and deseeded)

2 teaspoons lemon juice

Directions:

Push the ingredients through the juicer and juice.

Coco Berry Smoothie

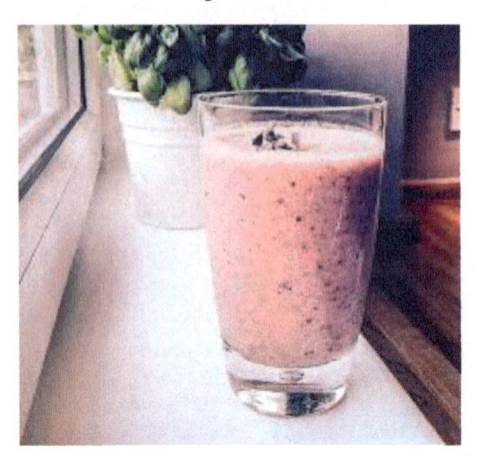

Preparation Time: 10 minutes

Servings: 4

Ingredients:

1 cupful of greens

1 cupful of water

2 peaches (skinned and deseeded)

1 banana (preferably frozen)

½ a cupful of wolfberries

½ a cupful of coconut flesh (diced)

Directions:

Put leafy greens and water in a pitcher and blend until the mix becomes a consistent green. Discontinue blending and put in residual ingredients. Turn on again and blend till it purees.

Cardiovascular Health Almond Cinnamon Smoothie

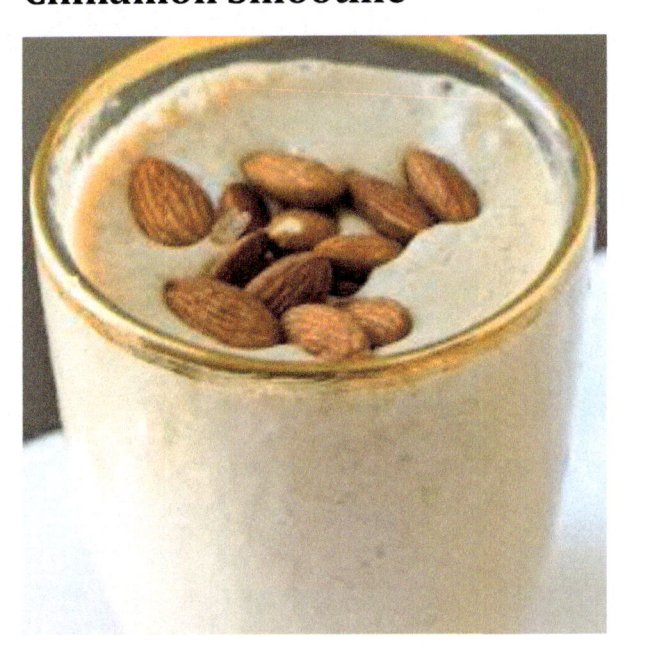

Preparation Time: 10 minutes

Servings: 4

Ingredients:

1 cupful of mesclun greens

1½ cupsful of almond milk

2 bananas

½ a teaspoonful of cinnamon

Directions:

Put leafy greens and water in a pitcher and blend until the mix becomes a consistent green.

Discontinue blending and put in residual ingredients. Turn on again and blend till it purees.

Oily Citrus Smoothie

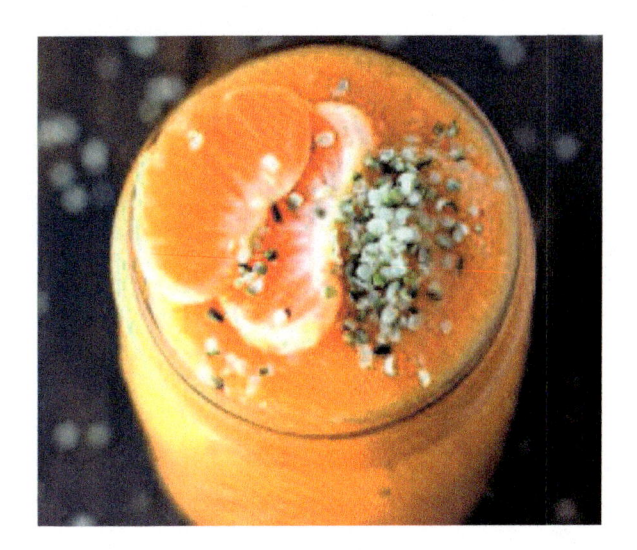

Preparation Time: 20 minutes

Servings: 4

Ingredients:

1 cupful of baby spinach

1 cupful of water

2 oranges (peeled and deseeded)

1 cupful of red grapes

2 tablespoons of ground flaxseeds

2 tablespoons of sunflower oil

Directions:

Put leafy greens and water in a pitcher and blend until the mix becomes a consistent green.

Discontinue blending and put in residual ingredients. Turn on again and blend till it purees.

The Medley of Romaine and Orange Juice

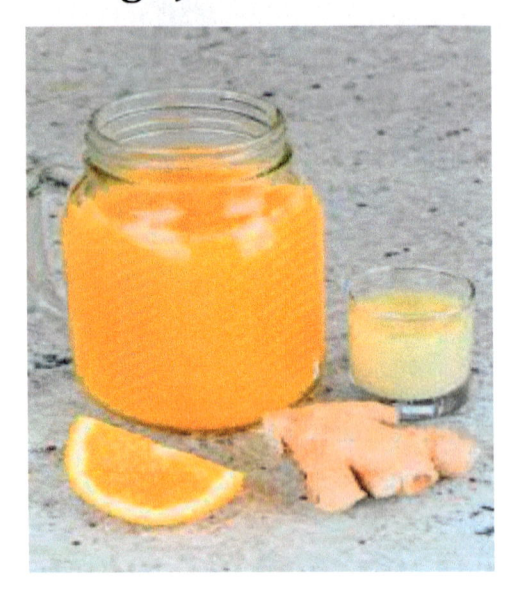

Preparation Time: 15 minutes

Servings: 3

Ingredients:

2 medium apples of 3-inch diameter

2 stalks of large celery

½ of a large cucumber

2 cups of romaine lettuce

1 peeled orange

Directions:

Add the ingredients to your juicer or centrifuge.

Process them thoroughly until you have a smooth juice.

Pour the drink into a glass and give it a nice shake.

Chill and serve!

Greasy Mango Smoothie

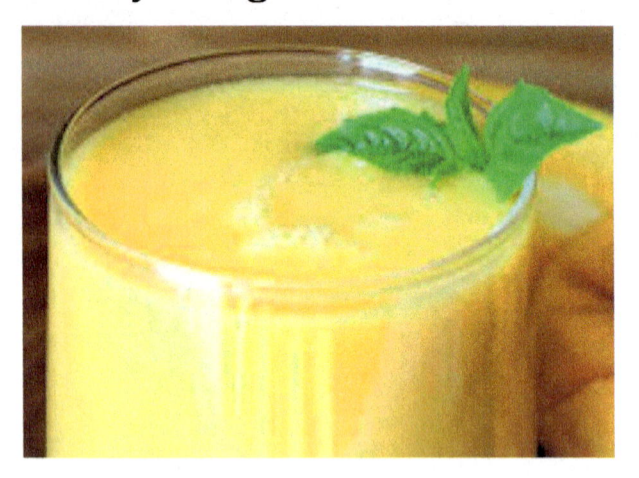

Preparation Time: 10 minutes

Servings: 4

Ingredients:

1 cupful of greens

1½ cupsful of almond/coconut milk

1½ cupsful of mango chunks (frozen)

1 banana

1 tablespoonful of extra-light olive oil

Directions:

Put leafy greens and water in a pitcher and blend until the mix becomes a consistent green.

Discontinue blending and put in residual ingredients. Turn on again and blend till it purees.

Berry Pastiche Smoothie

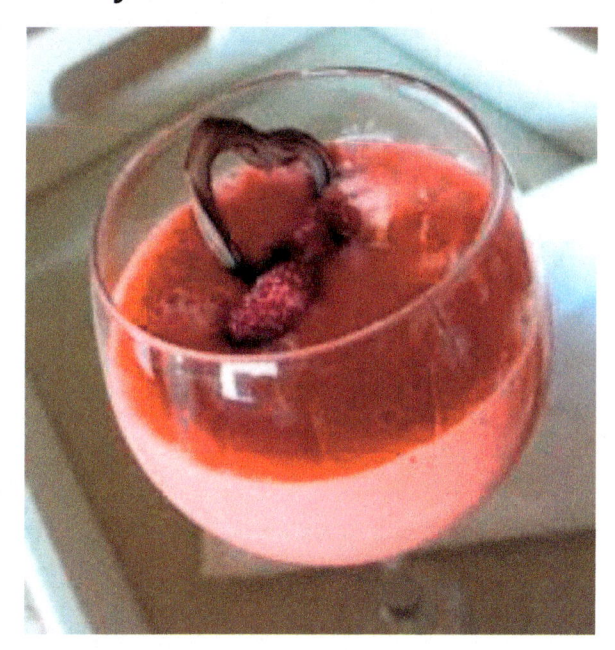

Preparation Time: 15 minutes

Servings: 4

Ingredients:

1 cupful of mixed greens

1½ cupsful of water

1 banana

2 cupsful of mixed berries (frozen)

2 tablespoons of flaxseed (ground)

Directions:

Put leafy greens and water in a pitcher and blend until the mix becomes a consistent green.

Discontinue blending and put in residual ingredients. Turn on again and blend till it purees.

Citrus Avocado Smoothie

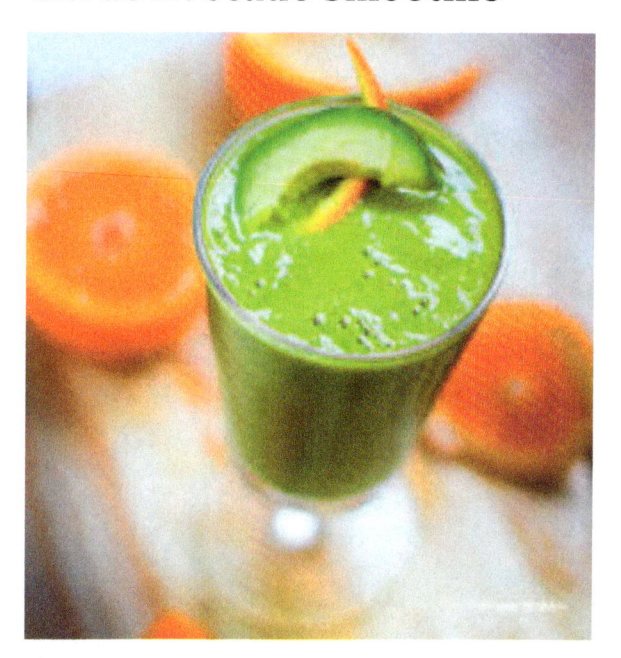

Preparation Time: 10 minutes

Servings: 3

Ingredients:

1 cupful of arugula

½ a cupful of ice

2 oranges (peeled and deseeded)

1 banana

½ an avocado

Directions:

Put leafy greens and water in a pitcher and blend until the mix becomes a consistent green.

Discontinue blending and put in residual ingredients. Turn on again and blend till it purees.

Carrot and Sweet Lime Juice

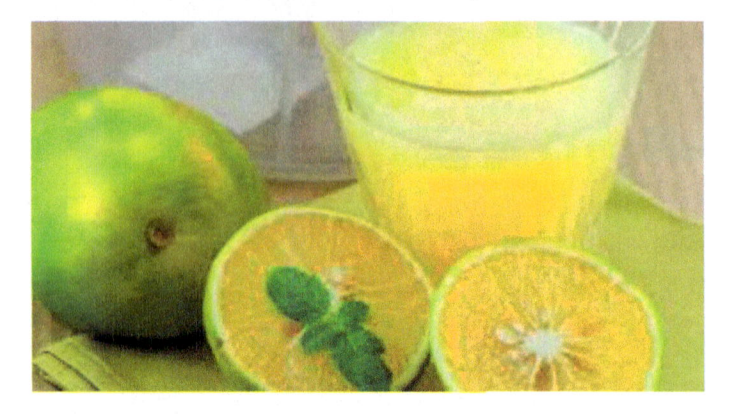

Preparation Time: 10 minutes

Servings: 3

Ingredients:

Boiled and cooled water

½ sweet lime

1 carrot

Directions:

Thoroughly wash the carrots, peel them then cut into small pieces; say an inch or 1 ½ inches.

Place the carrot pieces into a juicer and process them to obtain carrot juice. Make sure to dilute the juice with potable water particularly if introducing carrots to your kid's diet. A good ratio could be 3 parts water to 1-part carrot juice. Older children can have equal parts of water and juice.

Now add half of a sweet lime juice to the prepared carrot juice.

Dilute the juice as required then serve.

If need be, add in pureed raisins for extra sweetness.

The "Ginger" First Aid Juice

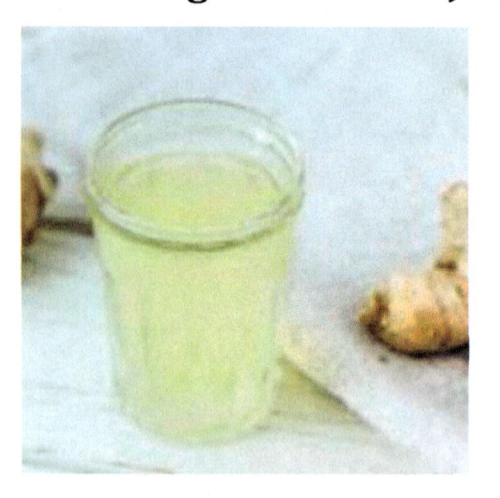

Preparation Time: 15 minutes

Servings: 3

Ingredients:

1 bunch of kale

½ a bunch of parsley

Green apple cut up into cubes and seeded

2-inch pieces of ginger

1 clove of garlic peeled

1 lemon fruit peeled

1 whole cucumber with ends discarded

Directions:

Add the ingredients to your juicer or centrifuge

Process them thoroughly until you have a smooth juice

Pour the drink into a glass and give it a nice shake

Chill and serve!

Radiantly Red Juice

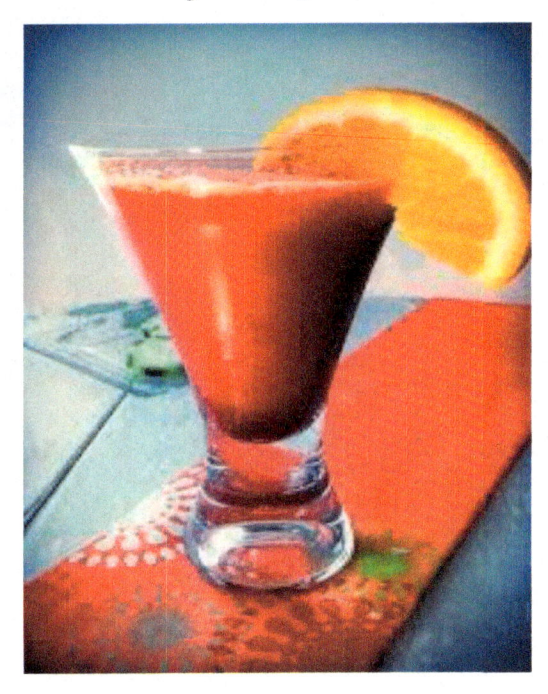

Preparation Time: 15 minutes

Servings: 4

Ingredients:

2 medium-sized apples

1 beet of a beetroot

4 medium-sized carrots

½ cucumber

1 cup of chopped dandelion greens

1 thumb of ginger root

2 kale leaves

2 peeled oranges

Directions:

Add the ingredients to your juicer or centrifuge.

Process them thoroughly until you have a smooth juice.

Pour the drink into a glass and give it a nice shake.

Chill and serve!

Green Celery Juice

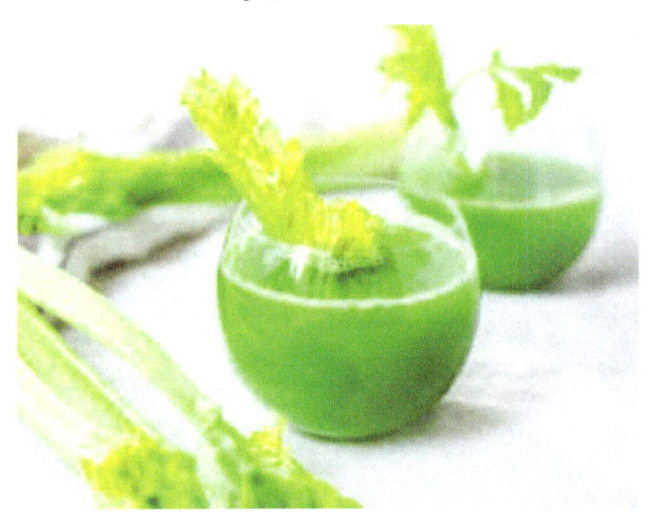

Preparation Time: 15 minutes

Servings: 4

Ingredients:

2 celery stalks

6 spinach leaves

1 handful parsley

4 carrots (peeled)

Directions:

Push all the ingredients through the juicer and juice.

Lemon "Get Up and Go" Smoothie

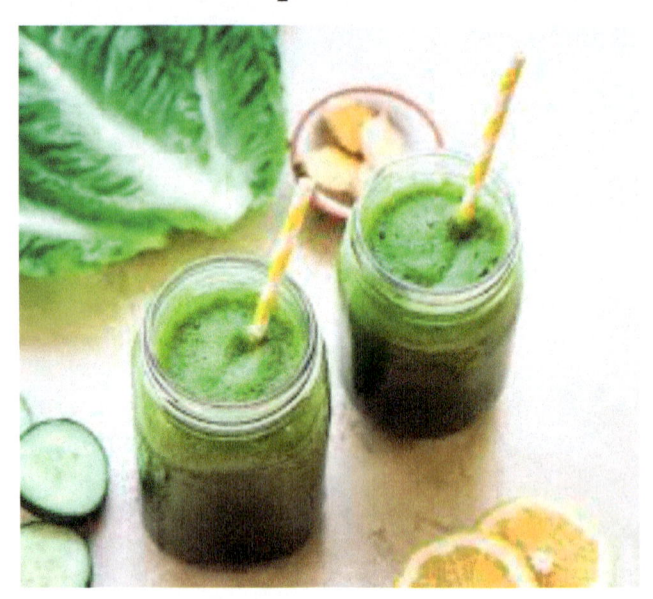

Preparation Time: 15 minutes

Servings: 4

Ingredients:

1 cupful of greens

1½ cupsful of orange juice (freshly squeezed)

1 cupful of ice

1 lemon (skinned)

1 tablespoon Methyl Sulfonyl Methane (MSM) powder

Directions:

Put leafy greens and water in a pitcher and blend until the mix becomes a consistent green.

Discontinue blending and put in residual ingredients. Turn on again and blend till it purees.

The "Beet Goes On" Juice

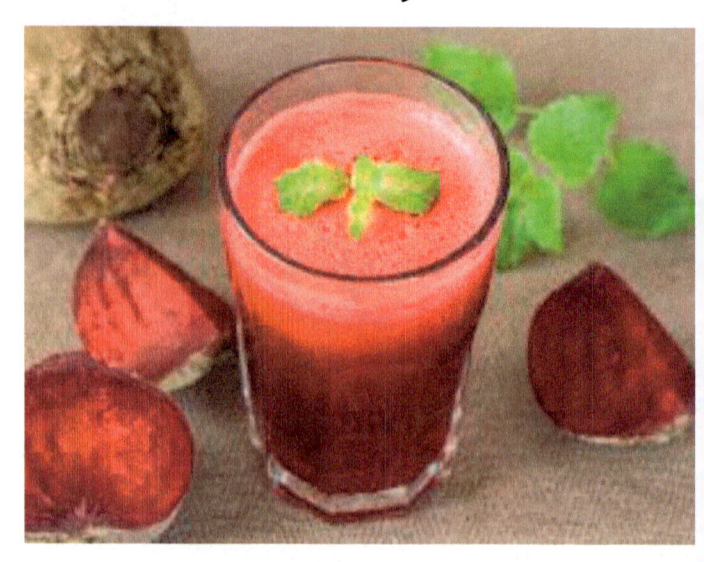

Preparation Time: 15 minutes

Servings: 4

Ingredients:

1 medium-sized apple of 3-inch diameter

1 beet of 2-inch diameter

3 medium-sized carrots

2 stalks of large celery

A handful of parsley

Directions:

Add the ingredients to your juicer or centrifuge

Process them thoroughly until you have a smooth juice

Pour the drink into a glass and give it a nice shake

Chill and serve!

Cabbage Cucumber Juice

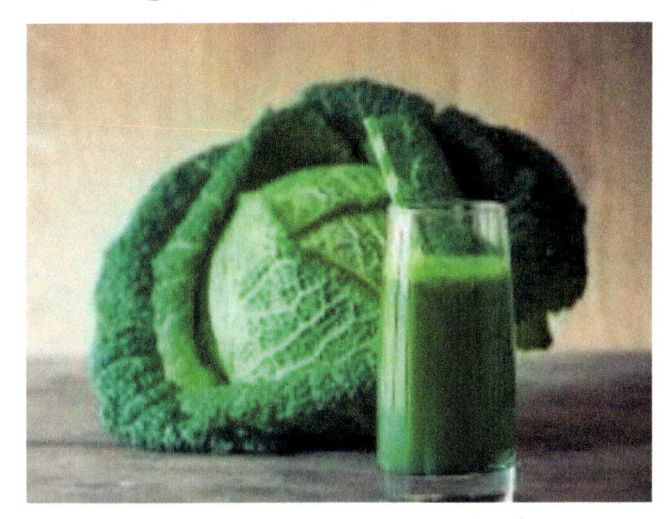

Preparation Time: 15 minutes

Servings: 4

Ingredients:

1/2 lemon juice

1 cup cucumber

1 cup cabbage

1/2 tsp salt

Directions:

Add all ingredients into the juicer and blend. Serve and enjoy.

Mint Grape Apple Juice

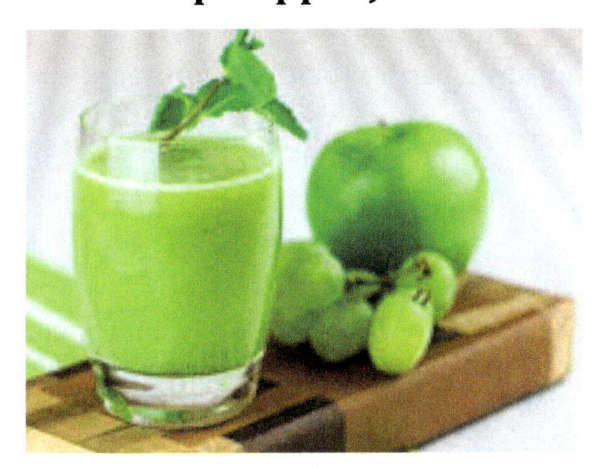

Preparation Time: 15 minutes

Servings: 4

Ingredients:

1 handful of fresh mint leaves

1 lime

5 green grapes

1/2-inch fresh ginger

1 medium apple

Directions:

Add all ingredients into the juicer and blend.

Serve and enjoy.

Super Delicious Fruit Juice

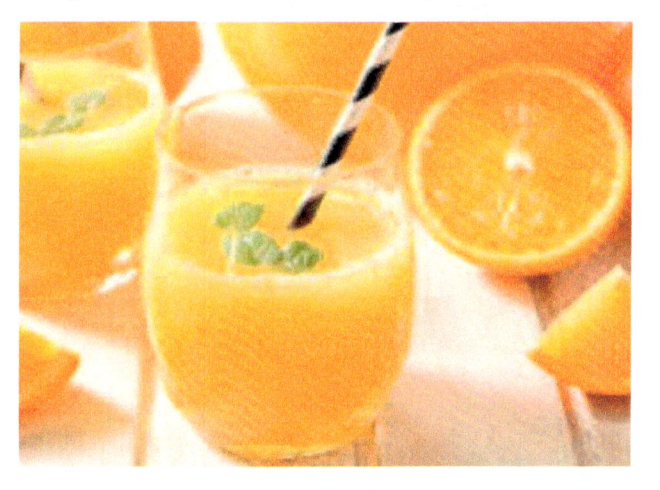

Preparation Time: 15 minutes

Servings: 4

Ingredients:

1/4 cup fresh coconut water

1 cup fresh pineapple

1/2 mango

1 orange

5 strawberries

1 kiwi, peeled

Directions:

Add all ingredients into the juicer and blend.

Serve immediately and enjoy.

Greenie Pear Smoothie

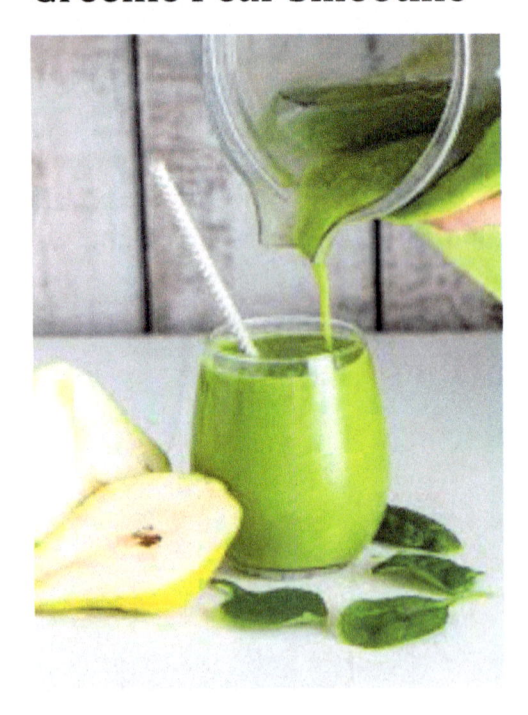

Preparation Time: 10 minutes

Servings: 4

Ingredients:

1 cupful of greens

1 cupful of water

1 pear

1 banana (peeled)

1 cupful of blueberries

Directions:

Put leafy greens and water in a pitcher and blend until the mix becomes a consistent green.

Discontinue blending and put in residual ingredients. Turn on again and blend till it purees.

Green Banana Smoothie

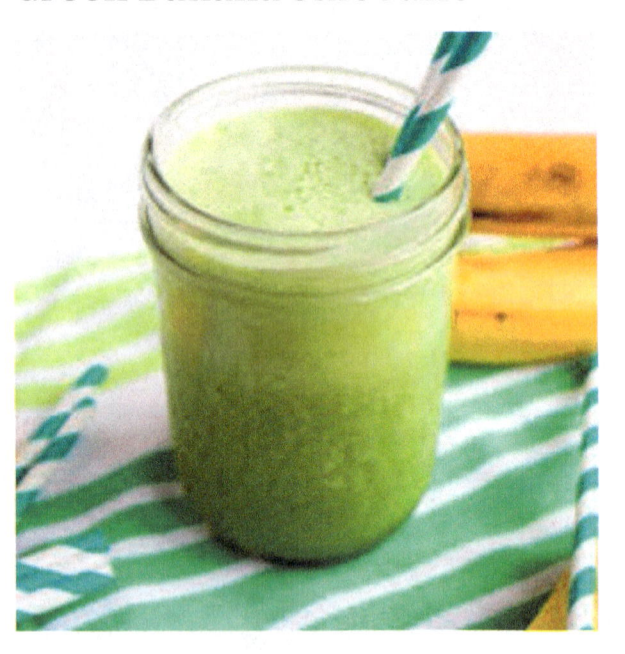

Preparation Time: 10 minutes

Servings: 4

Ingredients:

1 cupful of greens

1 cupful of water

1 banana (peeled)

1 cupful of strawberries (preferably frozen)

1 grapefruit (peeled and deseeded)

1 pack of stevia

Directions:

Put leafy greens and water in a pitcher and blend until the mix becomes a consistent green.

Discontinue blending and put in residual ingredients. Turn on again and blend till it purees.

Flaxseed Greens Smoothie

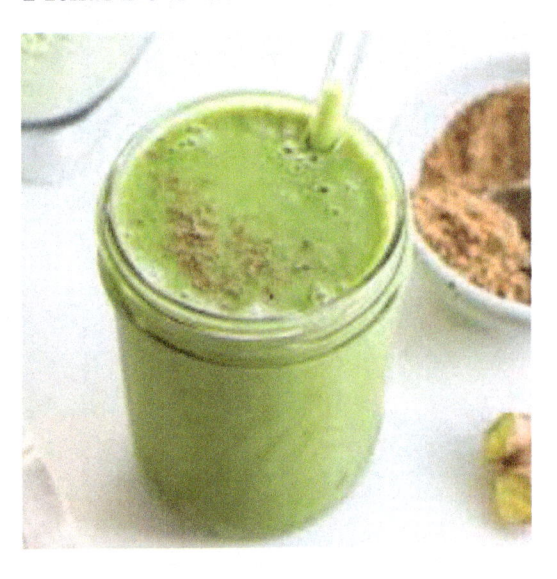

Preparation Time: 10 minutes

Servings: 4

Ingredients:

1 cupful of greens

1 cupful of water

1 frozen banana

1½ cupsful of blueberries

2 tablespoons of ground flaxseeds

Directions:

Put leafy greens and water in a pitcher and blend until the mix becomes a consistent green.

Discontinue blending and put in residual ingredients. Turn on again and blend till it purees.

Strawberry Greens Smoothie

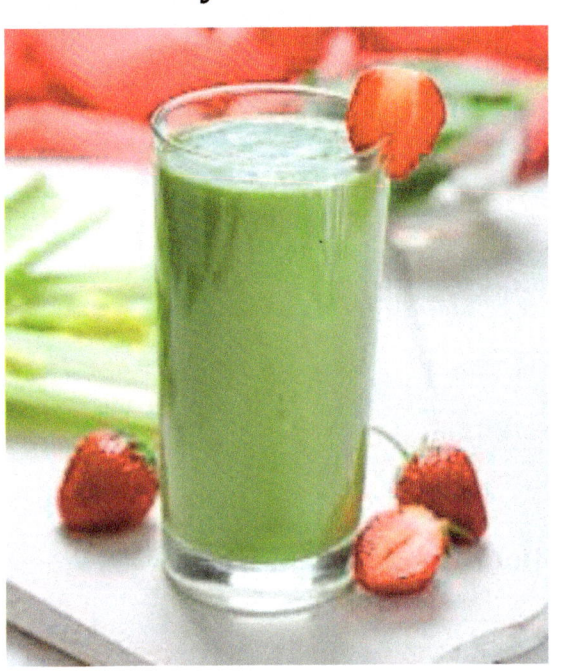

Preparation Time: 10 minutes

Servings: 4

Ingredients:

1 cupful of mixed greens

1 cupful of ice

1 midsize banana

2 cupsful of strawberries

½ avocado

Directions:

Put leafy greens and water in a pitcher and blend until the mix becomes a consistent green.

Discontinue blending and put in residual ingredients. Turn on again and blend till it purees.

Enlivener Citrus Pear Smoothie

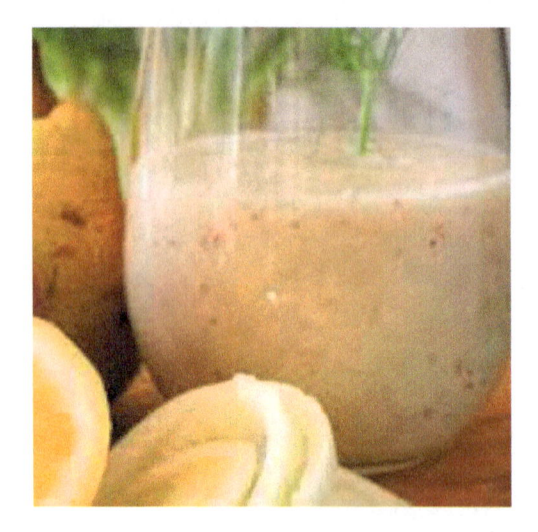

Preparation Time: 10 minutes

Servings: 4

Ingredients:

1 cupful of greens

½ cupful of ice

1 pear (cored and deseeded)

2 oranges (skinned and deseeded)

1 tablespoonful of flaxseeds (ground)

Directions:

Put leafy greens and water in a pitcher and blend until the mix becomes a consistent green.

Discontinue blending and put in residual ingredients. Turn on again and blend till it purees.

Avocado Berry Smoothie

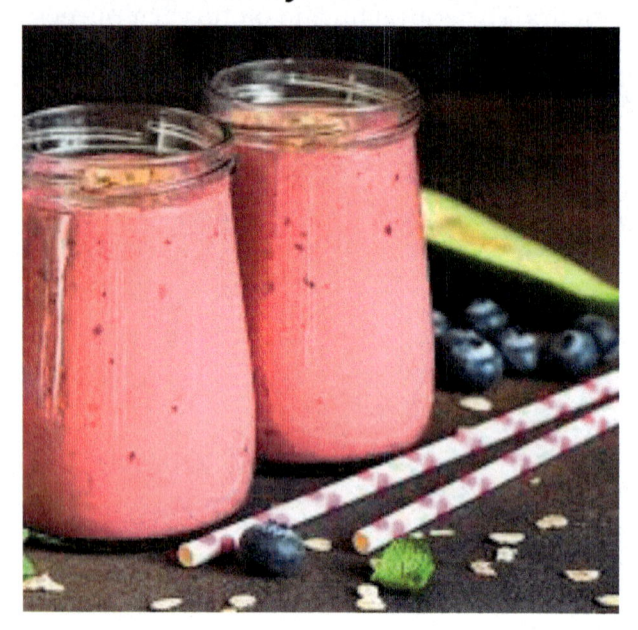

Preparation Time: 15 minutes

Servings: 4

Ingredients:

1 cupful of arugula

1 cupful of water

1½ cupsful of peaches (preferably frozen)

1 cupful of fresh mixed berries

1 small avocado (peeled and pitted)

Directions:

Put leafy greens and water in a pitcher and blend until the mix becomes a consistent green.

Discontinue blending and put in residual ingredients. Turn on again and blend till it purees.

Refreshing Lemon Berry Juice

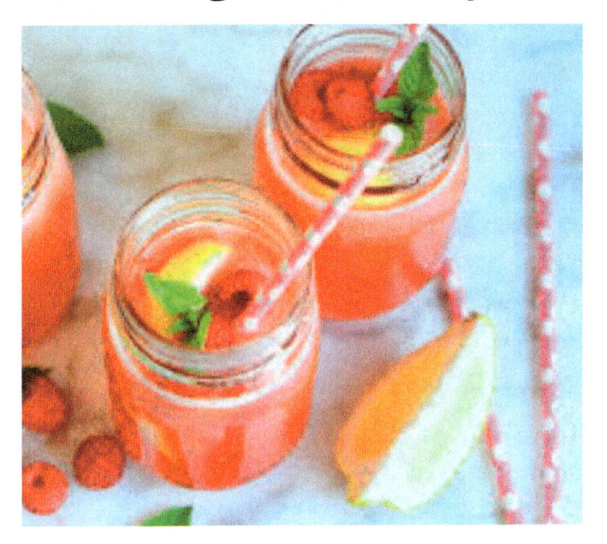

Preparation Time: 15 minutes

Servings: 4

Ingredients:

2 large carrots

1 cup raspberries

1 medium apple

1/2 orange, peeled

1/2 lime, peeled

1/2 lemon, peeled

1/2 head romaine lettuce

1/2 cucumber

Directions:

Add all ingredients into the juicer and blend.

Serve immediately and enjoy.

Passion Fruit Plum Juice

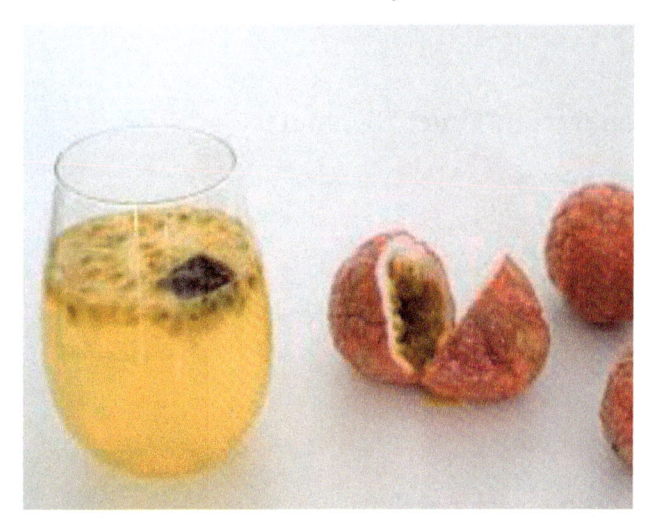

Preparation Time: 15 minutes

Servings: 4

Ingredients:

1 passion fruit

2 plums

1/8 tsp salt

1/2 tsp fennel seed powder

1/4 cup ice cubes

Directions:

Add all ingredients into the juicer and blend.

Serve and enjoy.

Healthy Coconut Oil Green Juice

Preparation Time: 15 minutes

Servings: 4

Ingredients:

1-inch fresh ginger

1 fresh lemon

1 fresh lime

1 handful fresh parsley

1 green apple

4 kale leaves

1 bunch celery

1 tbsp organic coconut oil

Directions:

Add all ingredients into the juicer and blend.

Serve and enjoy.

Spicy Berry Juice

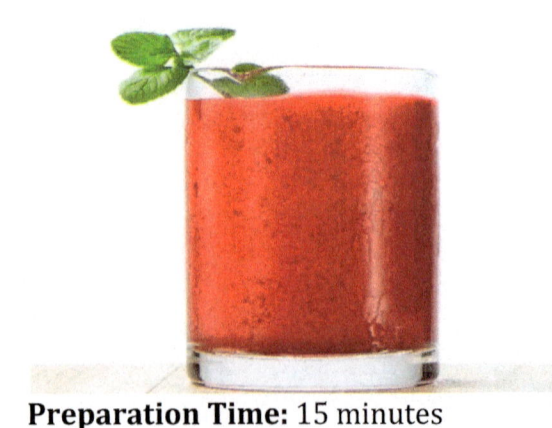

Preparation Time: 15 minutes

Servings: 4

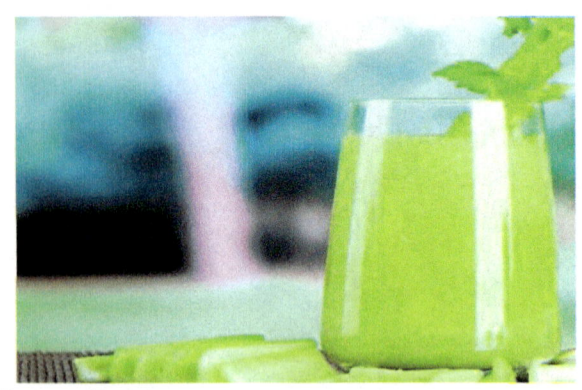

Ingredients:

1 small chili

1 cup fresh raspberries

1 cup dandelion leaves

2 cups fresh strawberries

Directions:

Add all ingredients into the juicer and blend.

Serve and enjoy.

Sweet and Spicy Mango Kale Juice

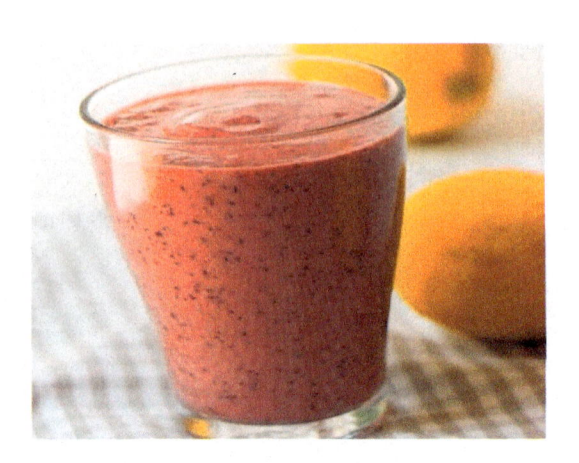

Preparation Time: 10 minutes

Servings: 4

Ingredients:

1 tbsp ground flaxseed

1/4 tsp cayenne pepper

1/4 avocado

1 tbsp lemon juice

1 cup kale

1/2 cup mango

1 cup fresh blueberries

1 1/2 cups coconut water

Directions:

Add all ingredients into the juicer and blend.

Serve and enjoy.

Refreshing Mint Kiwi Juice

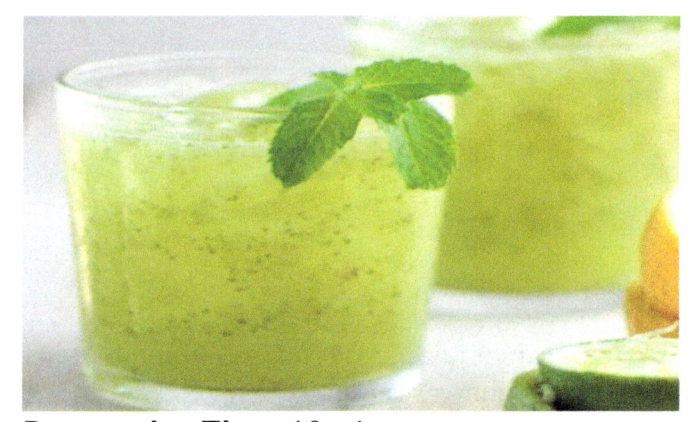

Preparation Time: 10 minutes

Servings: 4

Ingredients:

1 handful of fresh mint leaves

1/2 lime

1 cucumber

2 kiwis

Directions:

Add all ingredients into the juicer and blend. Serve and enjoy.

Red Bell Pepper Apple Juice

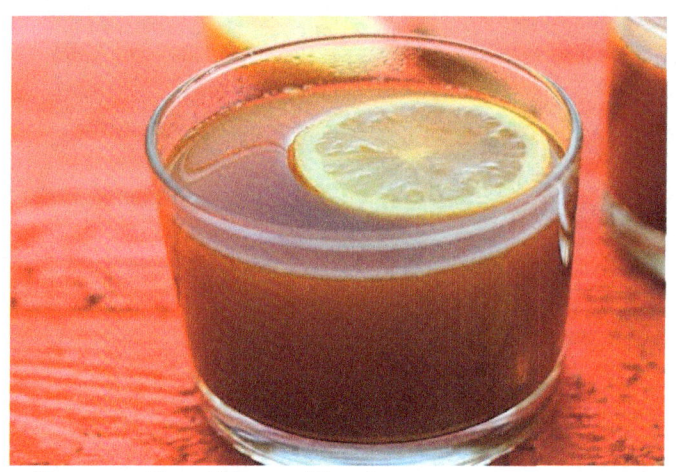

Preparation Time: 10 minutes

Servings: 4

Ingredients:

1 tbsp fresh lemon juice

1 medium apple

1 red bell pepper

Directions:

Add all ingredients into the juicer and blend.

Serve and enjoy.

Supreme Spinach Juice

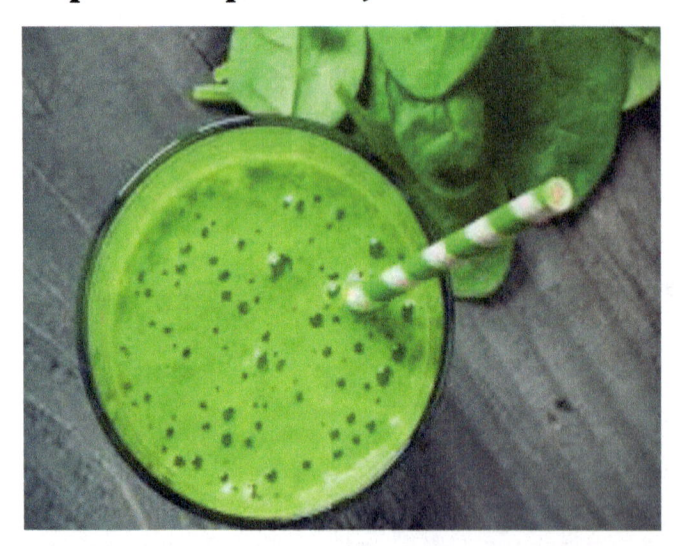

Preparation Time: 10 minutes

Servings: 4

Ingredients:

2 medium apples of 3-inch diameter

2 leaves of kale, each of 8-inch

A handful of kale

1 cup of spinach

Directions:

Add the ingredients to your juicer or centrifuge.

Process them thoroughly until you have a smooth juice.

Pour the drink into a glass and give it a nice shake. Chill and serve!

Pure Carrot juice

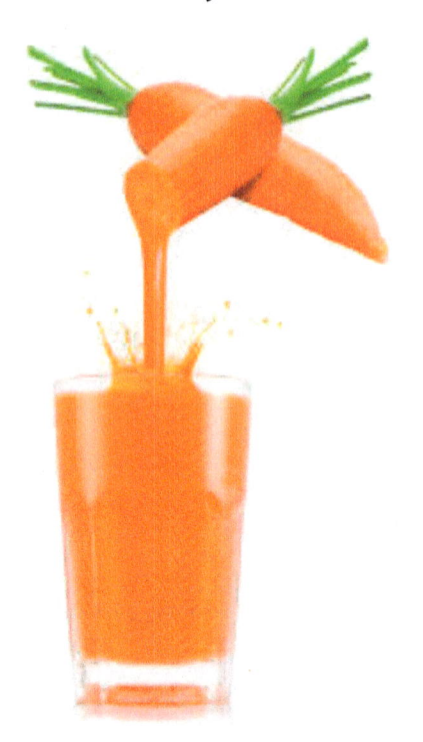

Preparation Time: 10 minutes

Servings: 3

Ingredients:

Boiled and cooled water

1 carrot

A few raisins, optional

Directions

Prepare carrot juice as described in the previous recipe and dilute as required.

Puree raisins that had been soaked in water overnight. Add the raisins to the juice to improve the taste.

Immunity Enhancer Greenie Strawberry Smoothie

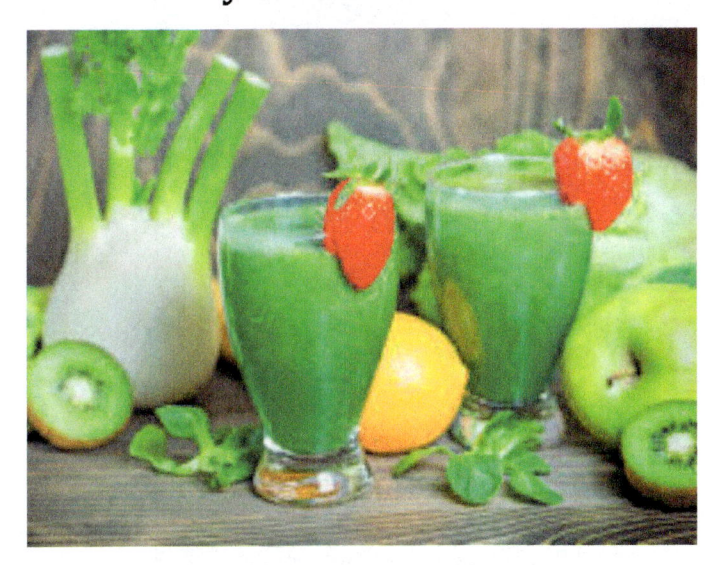

Preparation Time: 10 minutes

Servings: 4

Ingredients:

1 cupful of mixed greens

Juice of one lemon (freshly squeezed)

½ a cupful of frozen strawberries

1 banana

1 pack of stevia

Directions:

Put leafy greens and water in a pitcher and blend until the mix becomes a consistent green.

Discontinue blending and put in residual ingredients. Turn on again and blend till it purees.

Mango Berry Smoothie

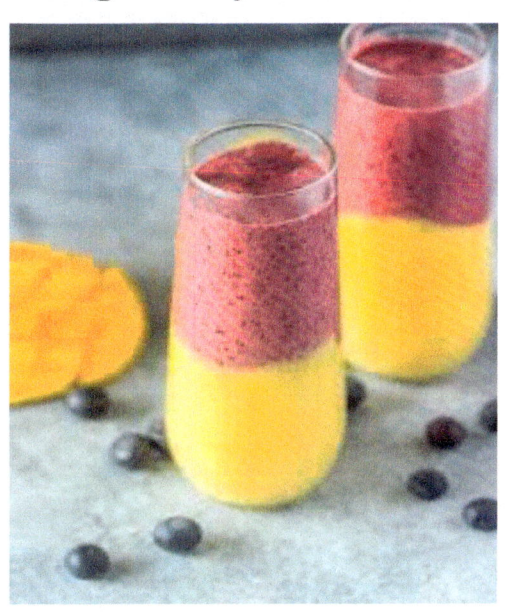

Preparation Time: 10 minutes

Servings: 4

Ingredients:

1 cupful of mesclun greens

1 cupful of water

½ a cupful of frozen blackberries

1 orange (skinned and deseeded)

½ a cupful of frozen raspberries

1 pack of stevia

1 cupful of frozen mango chunks

Directions:

Put leafy greens and water in a pitcher and blend until the mix becomes a consistent green.Discontinue blending and put in residual ingredients. Turn on again and blend till it purees.

Flaxy Banana Smoothie

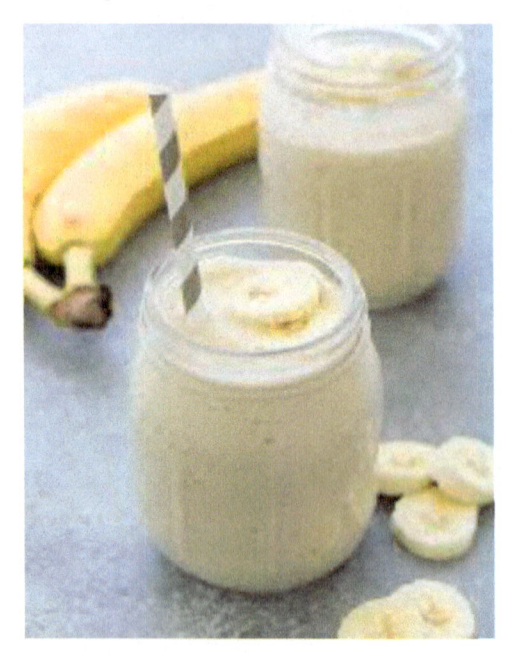

Preparation Time: 10 minutes

Servings: 4

Ingredients:

1 cupful of mesclun greens

1 cupful of water

1 banana

1½ a cupful of frozen blueberries

½ a cupful of ground flaxseeds

1 pack of stevia

Directions:

Put leafy greens and water in a pitcher and blend until the mix becomes a consistent green.

Discontinue blending and put in residual ingredients. Turn on again and blend till it purees.

Berry Greens Smoothie

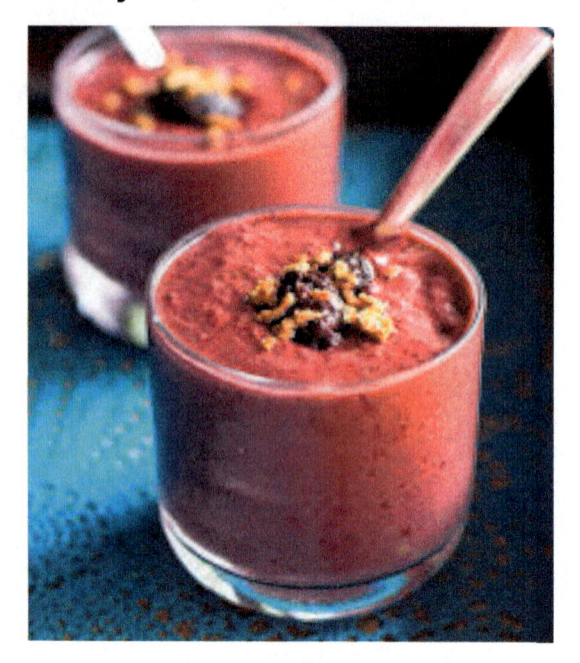

Preparation Time: 10 minutes

Servings: 4

Ingredients:

½ a cupful of greens

2 cupsful of coconut milk

1 banana (peeled and frozen)

½ a cupful of blueberries (frozen)

3 dates (pitted)

1 a cupful of blackberries (frozen)

Directions:

Put leafy greens and water in a pitcher and blend until the mix becomes a consistent green.

Discontinue blending and put in residual ingredients. Turn on again and blend till it purees.

The "Purple Yet Red" Juice

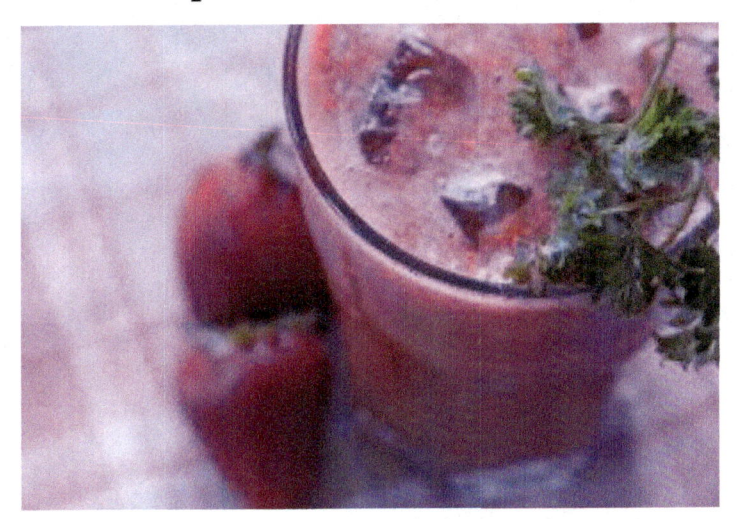

Preparation Time: 15 minutes

Servings: 4

Ingredients:

2 medium-sized apples of 3-inch diameter

2 red cabbage leaves

3 large carrots

1 cucumber of 8-inch length

1 peeled mango

1 and a ½ cup of whole strawberries

Directions:

Add the ingredients to your juicer or centrifuge.

Process them thoroughly until you have a smooth juice.

Pour the drink into a glass and give it a nice shake.

Chill and serve!

Tropical Fruit Juice

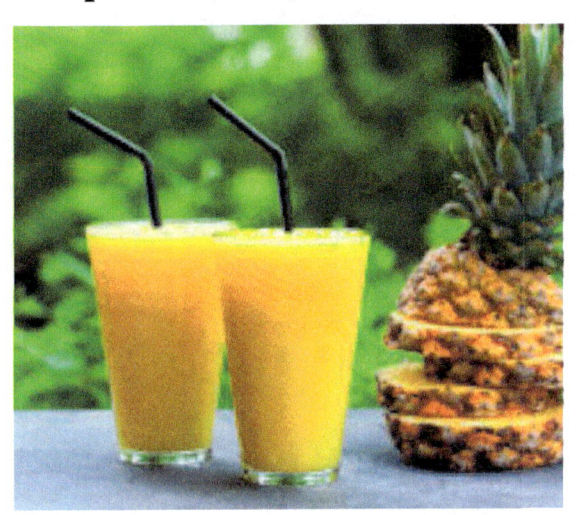

Preparation Time: 20 minutes

Servings: 3

Ingredients:

5 strawberries

1 slice of watermelon

1 slice of fresh pineapple

1/2 mango

1 orange

Directions:

Remove all the peels and seeds from the mango, watermelon, pineapple, and orange.

Add the peeled fruits to a juicer and process to get the juice.

Healthy Homemade Juice

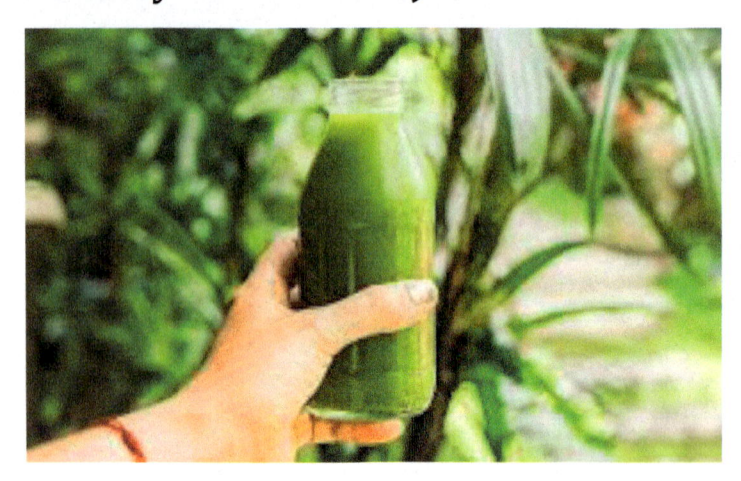

Preparation Time: 15 minutes

Servings: 3

Ingredients:

4-10 mint leaves (for flavor)

6 strawberries

Handful of blueberries

2 kiwis

2 apples

Directions:

Add all ingredients to a juicer.

Then process until ready and serve.

Minted Fruit Cocktail Juice

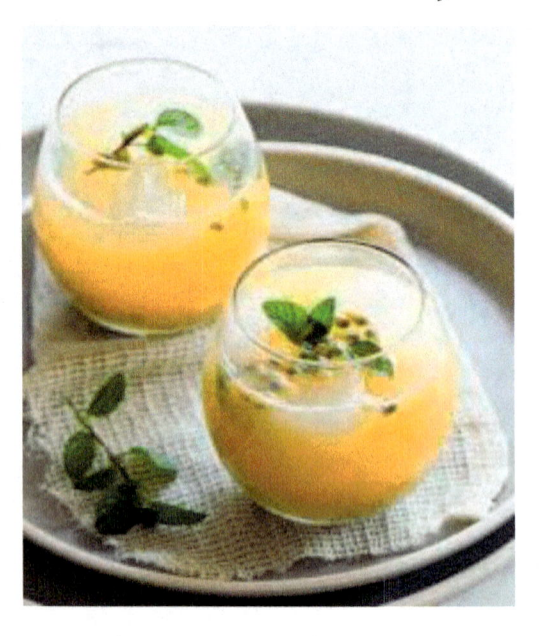

Preparation Time: 10 minutes

Servings: 3

Ingredients:

A small sprig of fresh mint

1 teaspoon lemon juice

2 cups watermelon, cubed and seeded

1/2 cup pineapple

1 orange, peeled and divided

1 apple, peeled, cored, and sliced

Directions:

Start by juicing the orange and the apple juice. Add in the pineapple.

Then add in mint, lemon juice, and watermelon, then juice.

Next, add in the apple-orange juice and then process until smooth. Serve

Chapter 5: Juices for Mental Health

Mango and Green Tea Juice

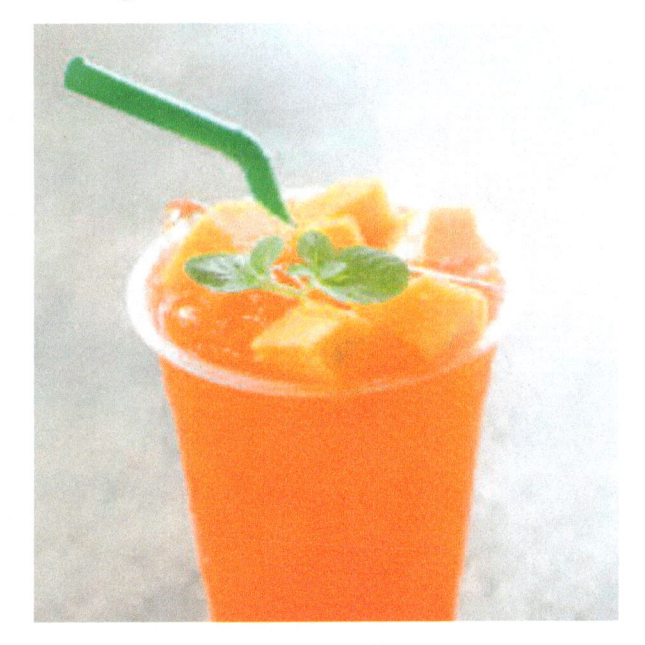

Preparation Time: 10 minutes

Servings: 3

Ingredients:

1 cup of mango, thinly sliced

½ cup of green tea, freshly brewed

1 tbsp. of honey

½ cup of low-fat yogurt

1 cup of ice cubes

Directions:

In a blender, add in the sliced mango, brewed green tea, honey, ice cubes, and low-fat yogurt.

Blend on the highest setting until smooth in consistency.

Pour into a chilled glass and serve immediately.

Apple, Red Leaf Lettuce, and Cucumber Juice

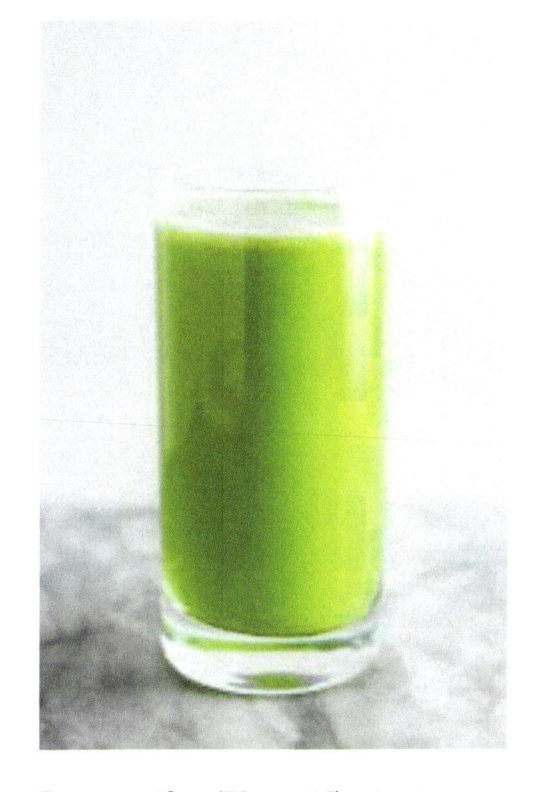

Preparation Time: 15 minutes

Servings: 3

Ingredients:

1 green apple, cored removed

½ of a lemon fruit

5 leaves of red leaf lettuce

1 cucumber, thinly sliced

Directions:

Wash the green apple, lemon fruits, leaves of red leaf lettuce, and cucumber thoroughly.

Peel the lemon fruit and remove the seeds 3. In a blender, add in the green apple, lemon fruit, red leaf lettuce, and sliced cucumber.

Blend on the highest setting until smooth in consistency. Pour into a chilled glass and serve immediately.

Cucumber and Apple Juice

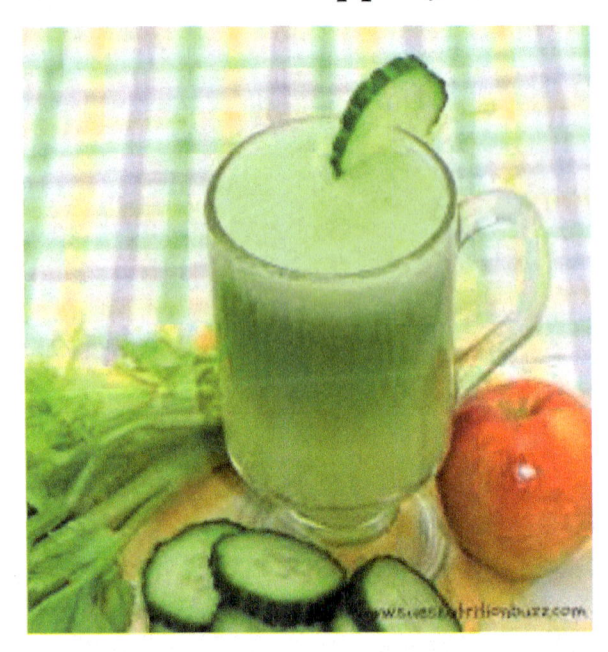

Preparation Time: 15 minutes

Servings: 3

Ingredients:

1 cucumber

1 apple

1 lemon wedge

1 cup mint leaves

Directions:

Add all the ingredients to the juicer and juice.

Papaya, Apple, and Dates Juice

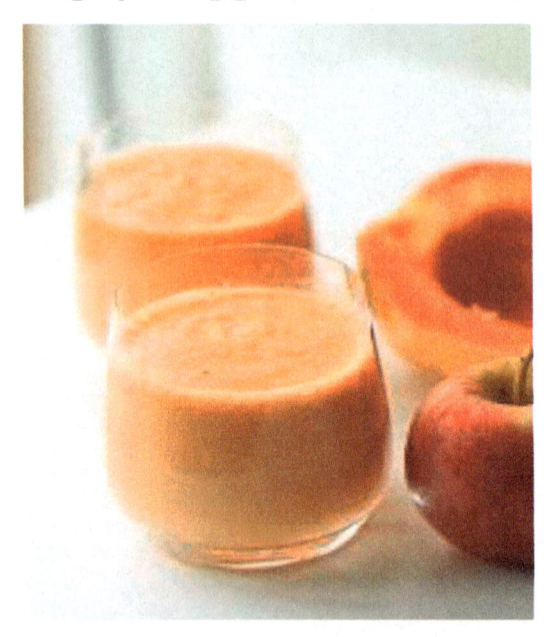

Preparation Time: 15 minutes

Servings: 3

Ingredients:

1 papaya

1 red apple, whole

5 dates, pits removed, and whole

Directions:

Wash the papaya and remove the seeds. Slice into 2-inch-thick slices.

Wash the dates thoroughly and slice into halves.

In a blender, add in the slices of papaya, red apple, and date halves.

Blend on the highest setting until smooth in consistency.

Pour into a chilled glass and serve immediately.

Apple, Kiwi, Pineapple, and Orange Juice

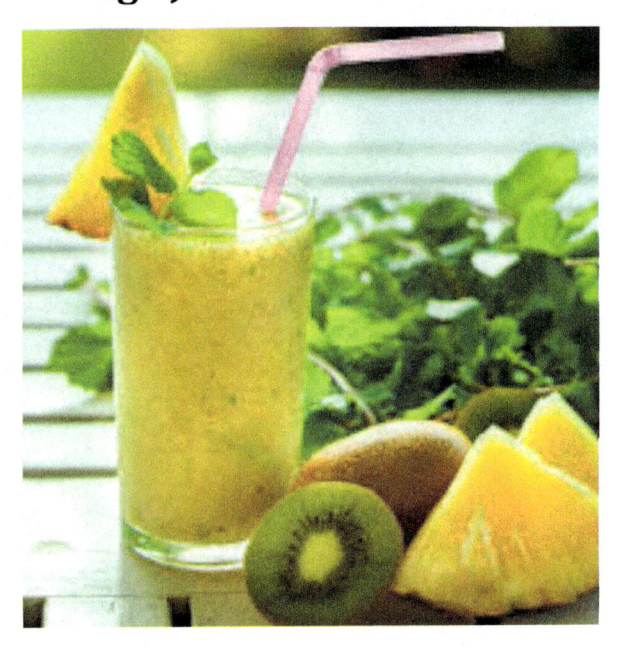

Preparation Time: 15 minutes

Servings: 3

Ingredients:

2 red apples

4 kiwis, whole

2 oranges, seedless

1 pineapple

Directions:

Remove the core from the apples and slice into thin wedges.

Peel the skin from the kiwis. Slice into 1-inch-thick slices.

Remove the rind from the oranges, leaving the white part of the skin intact.

Peel the pineapple and remove the core. Slice into thin spears.

In a blender, add in the slices of papaya, red apple, and date halves.

Blend on the highest setting until smooth in consistency.

Pour into a chilled glass and serve immediately.

Green Grape and Pepper Juice

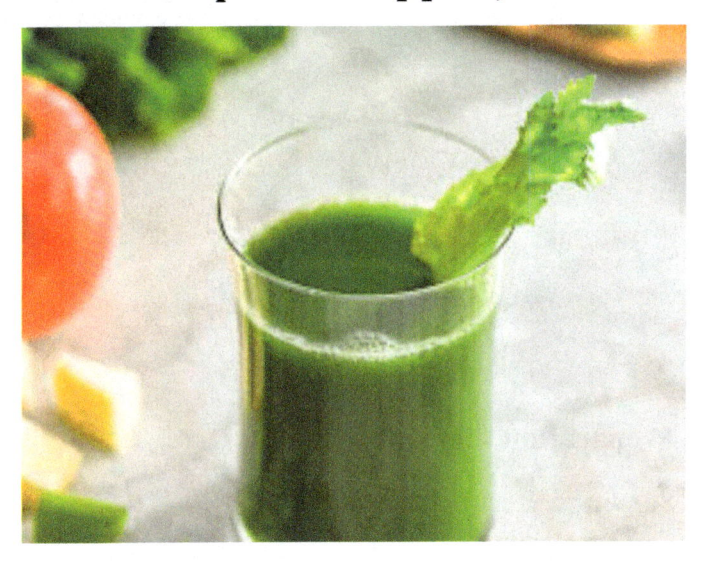

Preparation Time: 20 minutes

Servings: 3

Ingredients:

2 apples

3 carrots

1 bell pepper

1 cucumber

15 grapes

1 tomato

2 cups of spinach

Directions:

Add all the ingredients to the juicer and juice.

Strawberry Lime Juice

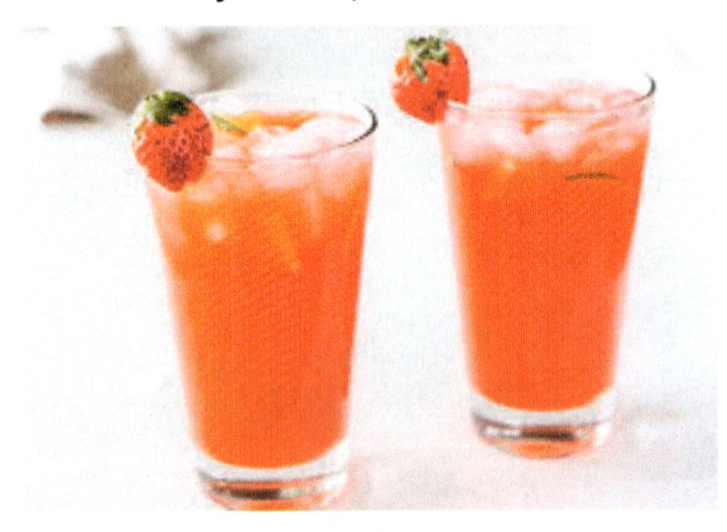

Preparation Time: 10 minutes

Servings: 3

Ingredients:

3 cups of strawberries

2 apples

½ Lime

Directions:

Add all the ingredients to the juicer and juice.

The Mind and Eye Opener Juice

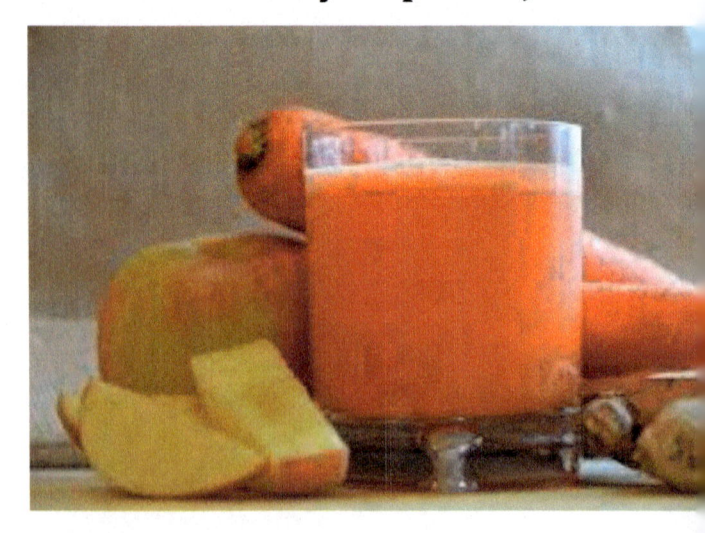

Preparation Time: 15 minutes

Servings: 2

Ingredients

2 medium-sized apples

14 medium-sized carrot

2 small-sized oranges

Directions:

Add the ingredients to your juicer or centrifuge.

Process them thoroughly until you have a smooth juice.

Pour the drink into a glass and give it a nice shake. Chill and serve!

Beetroot and Sweet Potato Juice

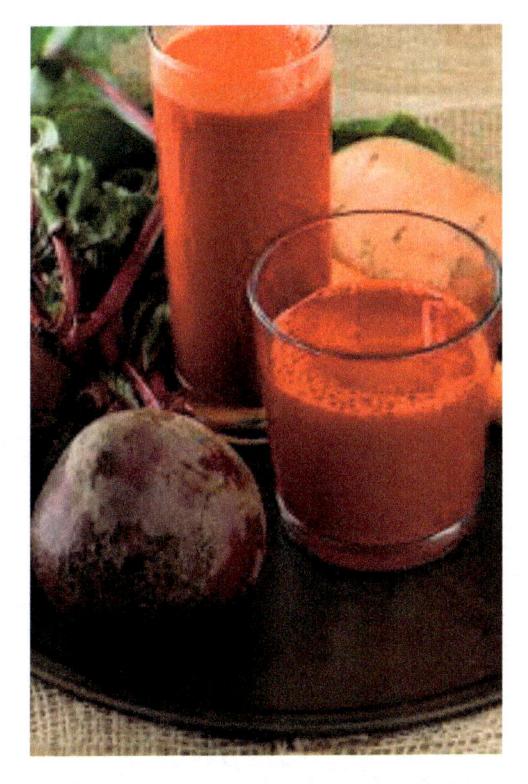

Preparation Time: 10 minutes

Servings: 3

Ingredients:

1 beetroot

1 sweet Potato

3 carrots

Directions:

Add all the ingredients to the juicer and juice.

Greens and Apple Juice

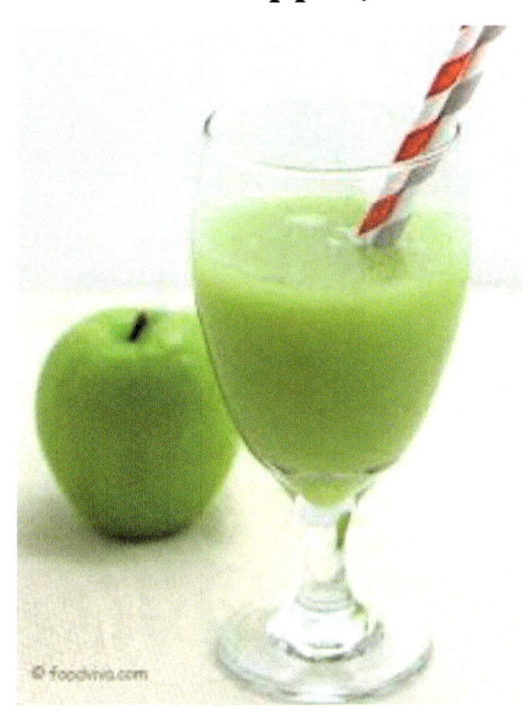

Preparation Time: 10 minutes

Servings: 3

Ingredients:

12 oz spinach

7 oz kale

6 oz golden apples

Directions:

Add all the ingredients to the juicer and juice.

Orange and Parsley Juice

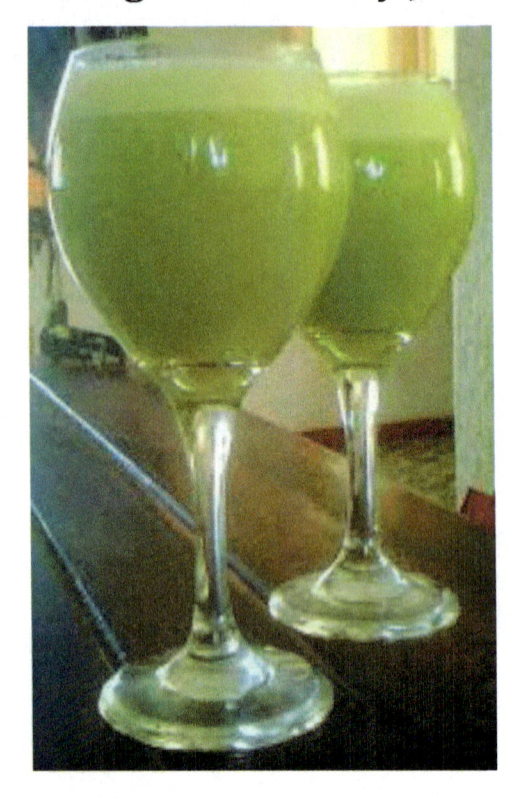

Preparation Time: 10 minutes

Servings: 3

Ingredients:

5 oranges, whole

½ cup of parsley, chopped

Directions:

Peel the oranges and remove the seeds.

Rinse the parsley under running water. Set aside to dry for 10 minutes.

In a blender, add in the oranges and chopped parsley.

Blend on the highest setting until smooth in consistency.

Pour into a chilled glass and serve immediately.

Muskmelon, Cactus, and Grape Juice

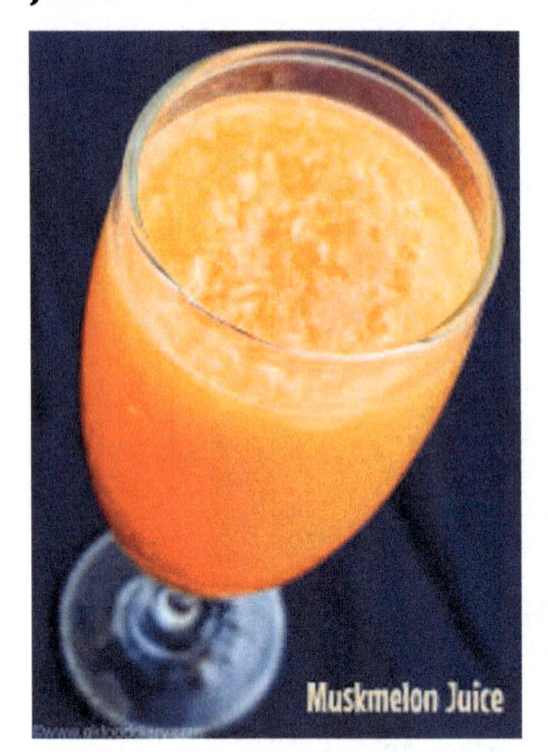

Preparation Time: 10 minutes

Servings: 3

Ingredients:

1 cup of grapes, seedless

¼ cup of cactus pear fruit juice

2 wedges of muskmelon

2 mangoes, whole

½ cup of ice cubes

Directions:

Wash the seedless grapes thoroughly.

Remove the skin and seeds from the muskmelon. Slice into 2-inch-thick slices.

Peel the skin from the mango and remove the inner seed. Slice into 2-inch-thick slices.

In a blender, add in the grapes, pear fruit juice, muskmelon slices, mango slices, and ice cubes.

Blend on the highest setting until smooth in consistency.

Pour into a chilled glass and serve immediately.

Salty and Sweet Pineapple Juice

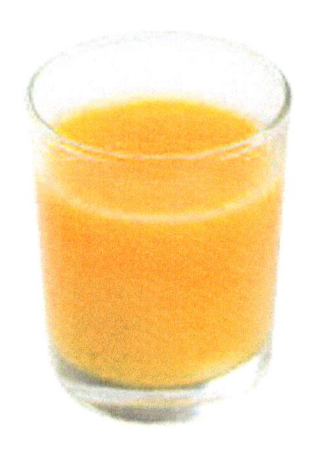

Preparation Time: 15 minutes

Servings: 3

Ingredients:

½ cup of pineapple chunks

2 Tbsp. of white sugar

¼ tsp. of salt

1 cup of water, filtered

Directions:

In a bowl, add in the white sugar and salt. Stir to mix. Add in the filtered water and stir well until dissolved.

Add the chunks of pineapple into the water mix. Set aside to soak for 10 minutes.

In a blender, add in the pineapple and water mix.

Blend on the highest setting until smooth in consistency. Pour into a chilled glass and serve immediately.

Pineapple, Watermelon, and Mango Juice

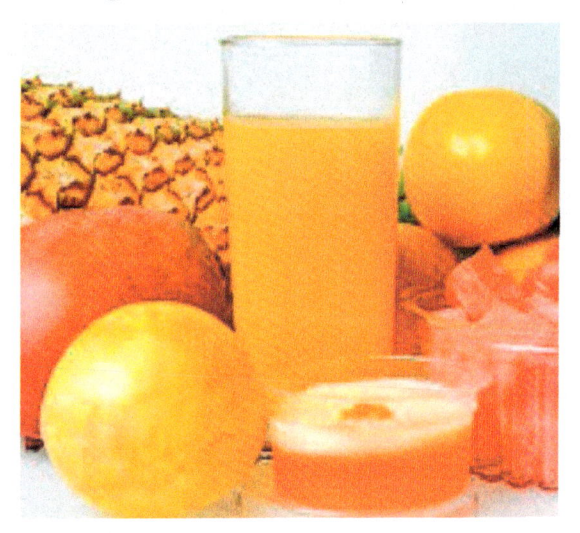

Preparation Time: 10 minutes

Servings: 3

Ingredients:

½ of a watermelon

1 mango, whole

1 ½ cups of pineapple, cut into chunks

Directions:

Remove the outer rind from the watermelon. Slice into 2-inch sized chunks.

Peel the mango and remove the seed from the inside. Slice into 2-inch-thick slices.

In a blender, add in the pineapple chunks, mango sliced and chunks of watermelon. 4. Blend on the highest setting until smooth in consistency.

Pour into a chilled glass and serve immediately.

Brain Booster Juice

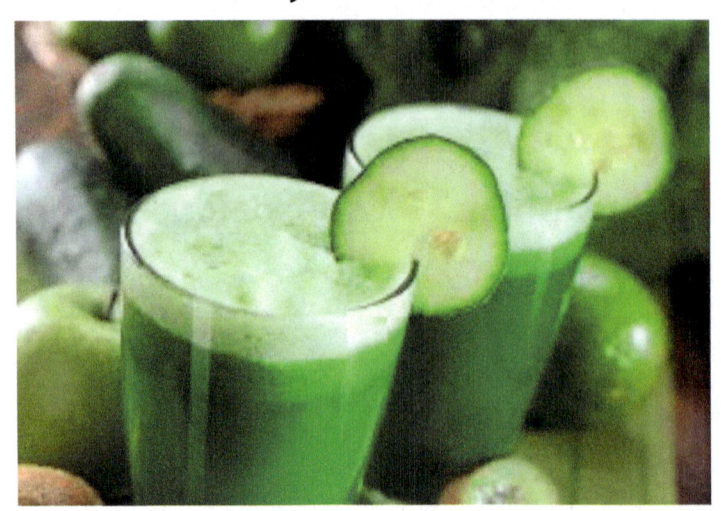

Preparation Time: 10 minutes

Servings: 3

Ingredients:

1 ½ cups carrot cubes

1 cup apple cubes –

¼ cup beetroot cubes

½ cup chopped spinach

Directions:

Add all the ingredients to the juicer and juice.

Chapter 6: Juices for Youthful Skin

Red Cabbage, Ginger, and Grape Juice

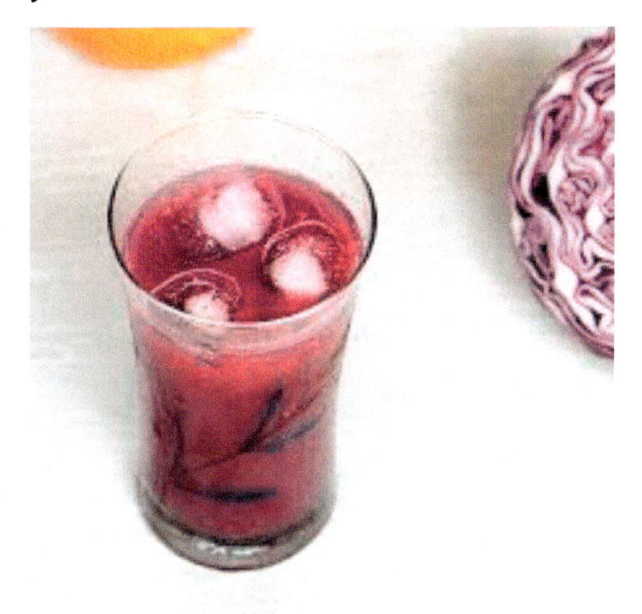

Preparation Time: 15 minutes

Servings: 3

Ingredients:

1 cup of grapes, seedless

1 1/3 cup of apples, core removed and chopped

¼ cup of red cabbage, chopped coarsely

3 stalks of celery

1, 3-inch piece of ginger

1 Tbsp. of balsamic vinegar

Directions:

Wash the seedless grapes, chopped apples, red cabbage, celery, and ginger thoroughly.

In a blender, add in the seedless grapes, chopped apples, chopped red cabbage, stalks of celery, ginger, and balsamic vinegar.

Blend on the highest setting until smooth in consistency.

Pour into a chilled glass and serve immediately.

Cucumber, Kale and Spinach Juice

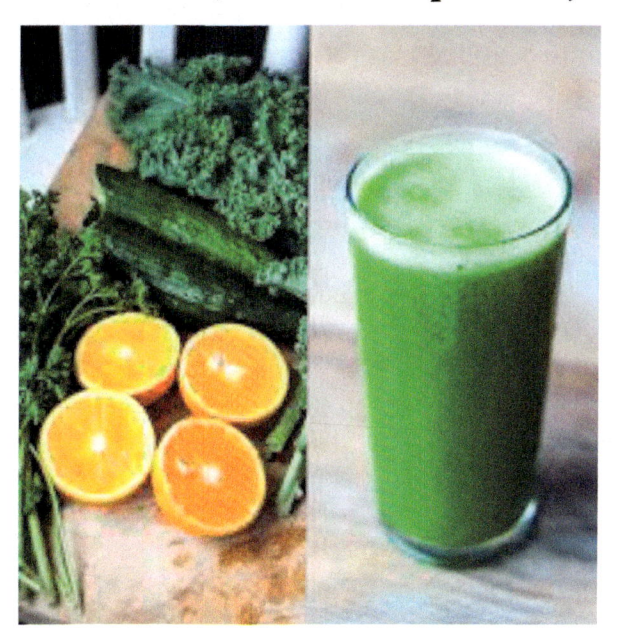

Preparation Time: 15 minutes

Servings: 3

Ingredients:

2 cucumbers, whole

½ cup of kale

¼ cup of spinach

¼ cup of parsley, chopped

¼ cup of Swiss chard

½ a slice of lemon

Directions:

Rinse the kale, spinach, chopped parsley, and Swiss chard thoroughly. Remove the steam. Wash the cucumber thoroughly. Slice into 1-inch-thick slices.

Remove the rind and seeds from the lemon. Slice into 1-inch-thick slices.

In a blender, add in the cucumbers, kale, spinach, chopped parsley, Swiss chard, and lemon slices.

Blend on the highest setting until smooth in consistency.

Pour into a chilled glass and serve immediately.

Bruschetta Juice

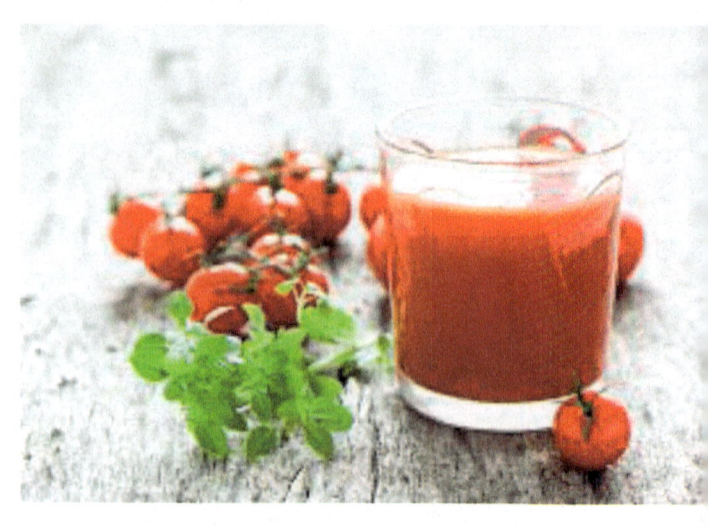

Preparation Time: 15 minutes

Servings: 3

Ingredients:

2 tomatoes

1-2 peeled garlic cloves

1 bunch of basil

¼ peeled lemon

2 celery stalks

Directions:

Combine all ingredients in the juicer. Serve immediately and enjoy or refrigerate. The juice will stay good in the refrigerator for up to 24 hours. This juice can also be served warm, making it perfect for those cold days.

Heavy Metal Detox Juice

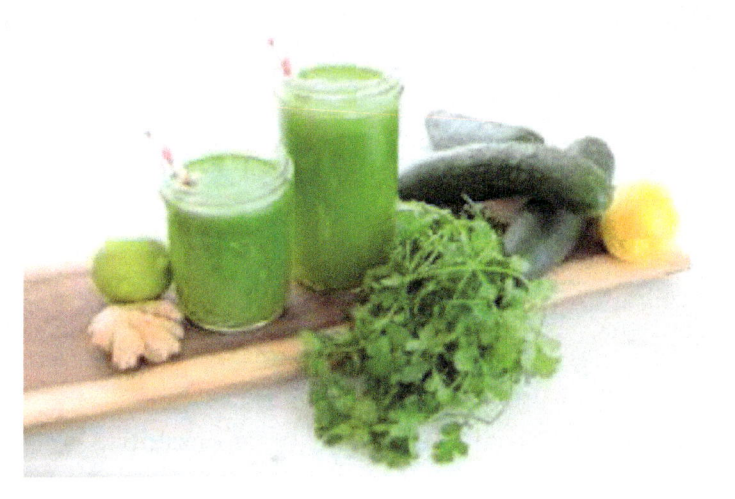

Preparation Time: 10 minutes

Servings: 3

Ingredients:

2 cups of pineapple

2 cored apples

1 lemon

2 cucumbers

6 stalks of celery

1 head of romaine

1 small bunch of cilantro

1 small bunch of mint

3 kale stalks

Directions:

Juice cucumbers, apples, lemon, and pineapple first followed by kale, Romain, cilantro, celery, and mint. Serve immediately and enjoy or refrigerate. The juice will stay good in the refrigerator for up to 24 hours.

Avocado, Spinach, and Lime Juice

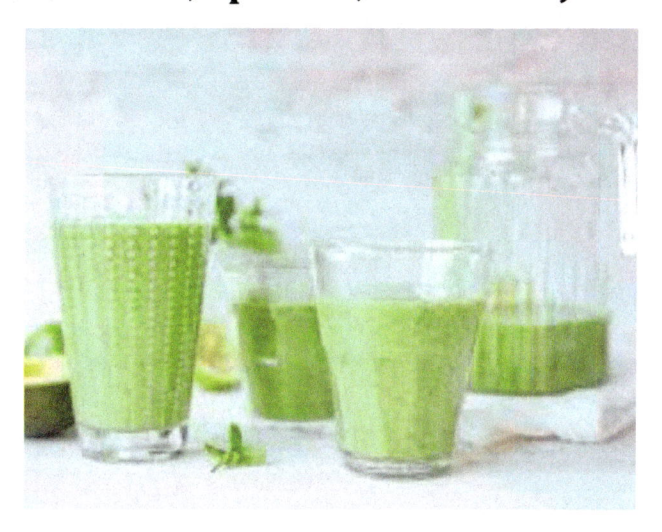

Preparation Time: 15 minutes

Servings: 4

Ingredients:

1 1/3 cup of avocado, cut into cubes

2/3 cup of grapes, seedless

2 apples, core removed

2 cups of spinach leaves

3 stalks of celery, chopped

1 lime fruit, cut into pieces

Directions:

Wash the avocado, seedless grapes, apple, spinach leaves, chopped celery, and lime fruit thoroughly.

Slice the avocado into halves and remove the seed.

Peel the lime and remove the seeds.

In a blender, add in the apples, seedless grapes, avocado cubes, spinach leaves, chopped stalks of celery, and lime fruit pieces.

Blend on the highest setting until smooth in consistency.

Pour into a chilled glass and serve immediately.

The Ultimate Skin Immune Booster Juice

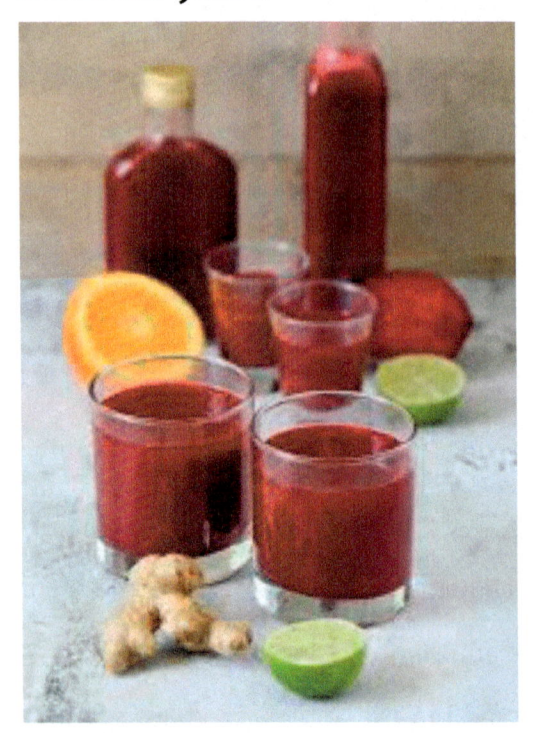

Preparation Time: 10 minutes

Servings: 4

Ingredients:

2 medium-sized apples of 3-inch diameter

7 medium carrots

2 cloves of garlic

1 ginger root thumb

A handful of parsley

Directions:

Add the ingredients to your juicer or centrifuge.

Process them thoroughly until you have a smooth juice.

Pour the drink into a glass and give it a nice shake.

Chill and serve!

Sunset Passion Juice

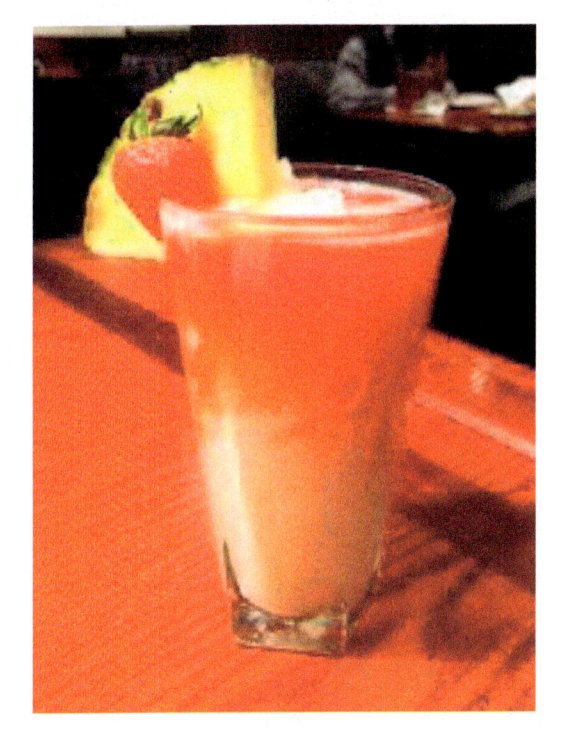

Preparation Time: 15 minutes

Servings: 3

Ingredients:

1 beet sliced

1 cucumber

1 carrot

1 Granny Smith apple

4 kale leaves

¼ peeled lemon

¼ peeled lime

Directions:

Juice beets, cucumber, apple, lemon, and lime followed by the kale leaves. Serve immediately and enjoy or refrigerate. The juice will stay good in the refrigerator for up to 24 hours.

Best Face Forward Juice

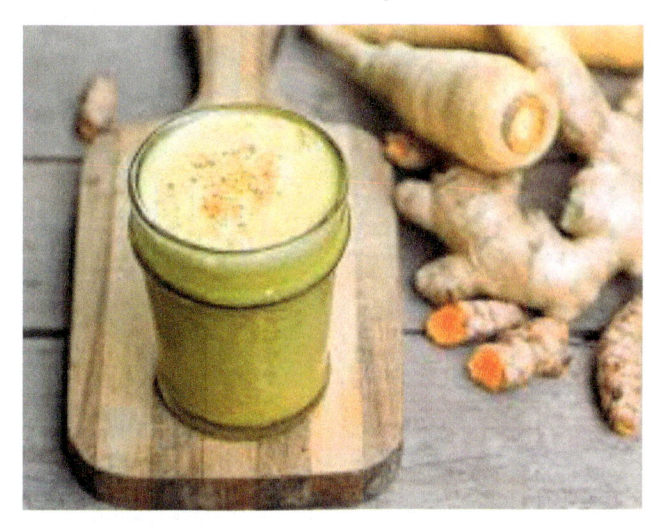

Preparation Time: 15 minutes

Servings: 3

Ingredients:

1 cucumber

1 parsnip

2-3 carrots

Half of a peeled lemon

¼ of a seeded green pepper

Directions:

Juice cucumber, parsnip, and carrots first, followed by green pepper and lemon. Serve immediately or refrigerate. The juice will stay good in the refrigerator for up to 24 hours.

Refreshing Renewal Juice

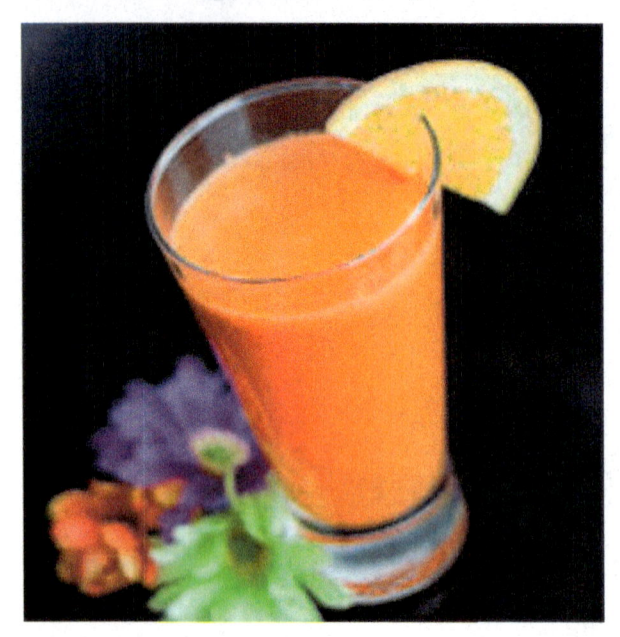

Preparation Time: 20 minutes

Servings: 3

Ingredients:

2 stalks of fennel

Half of a cucumber

Half of a cored green apple

1 handful of mint

1 inch of ginger root

Directions:

Juice all ingredients. Serve immediately and or refrigerate. The juice will stay good in the refrigerator for up to 24 hours.

Ultimate Veggie Mix Juice

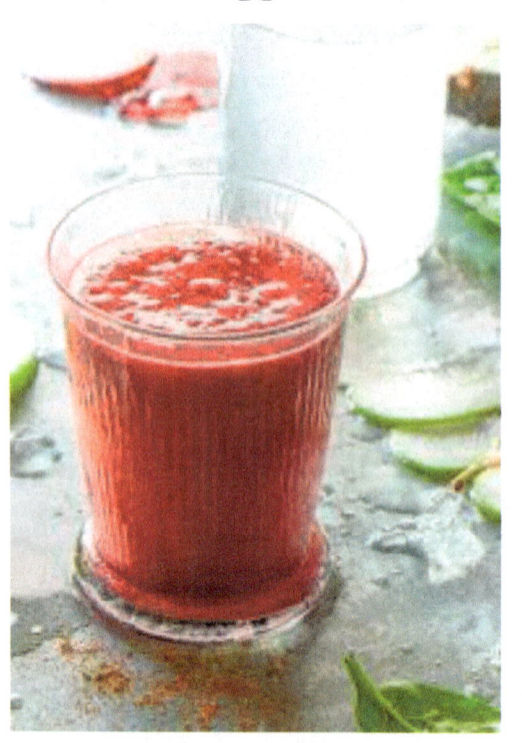

Preparation Time: 10 minutes

Servings: 3

Ingredients:

1 cucumber

3 carrots

1 beet

2 stalks of celery

1 handful of parsley

Half a peeled lemon

Directions:

Juice all ingredients. Serve immediately and or refrigerate. The juice will stay good in the refrigerator for up to 24 hours.

The Green Cucumber Juice

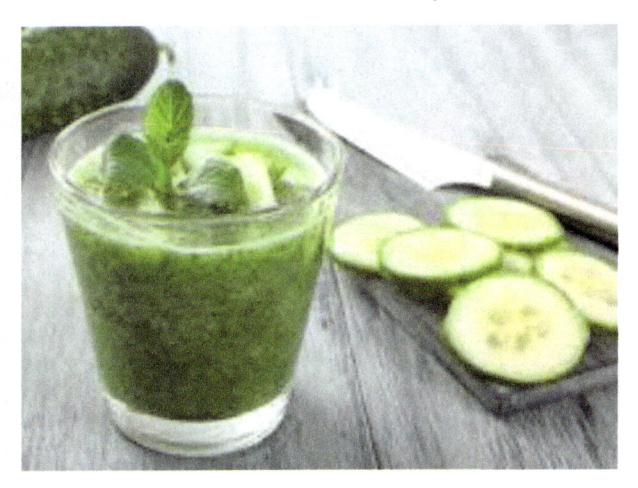

Preparation Time: 10 minutes

Servings: 3

Ingredients:

1 cucumber

1 large cup of spinach

1 large cup of parsley

1 celery stock

½ of a peeled lemon

Directions:

Combine all ingredients in the juicer. Serve immediately or refrigerate. The juice will stay good in the refrigerator for up to 24 hours.

Pink Delight Juice

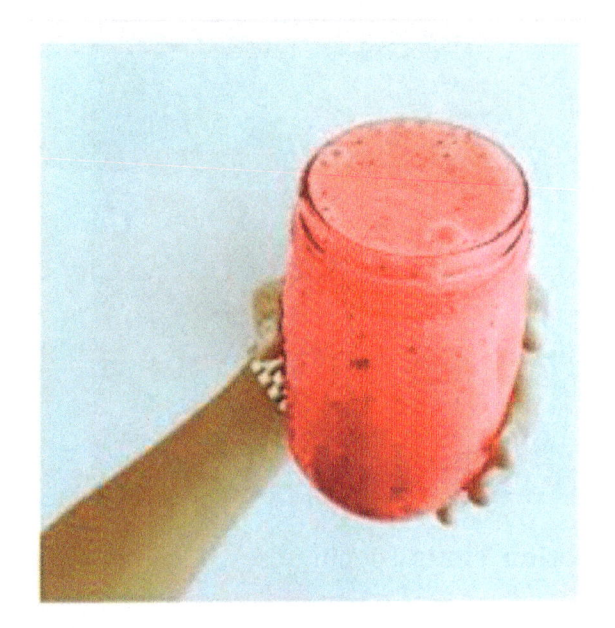

Preparation Time: 10 minutes

Servings: 3

Ingredients:

8 oz. of watermelon

4 oz. of strawberries

4 oz. of raspberries

½ cup sparkling water (optional)

Directions:

Combine the fruits in the juicer. Add sparkling water for a little fizz if desired. Serve immediately or refrigerate. The juice will stay good in the refrigerator for up to 24 hours.

Ginger Root Boost Juice

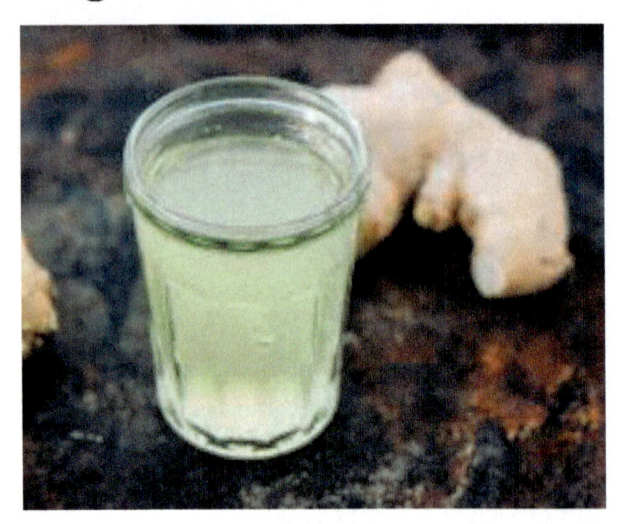

Preparation Time: 10 minutes

Servings: 3

Ingredients:

1 inch of ginger

1 peeled lemon

6 carrots (green tops optional)

1 cored apple

Directions:

Combine all ingredients in the juicer. Serve immediately or refrigerate. The juice will stay good in the refrigerator for up to 24 hours.

Ginger-Watermelon Juice

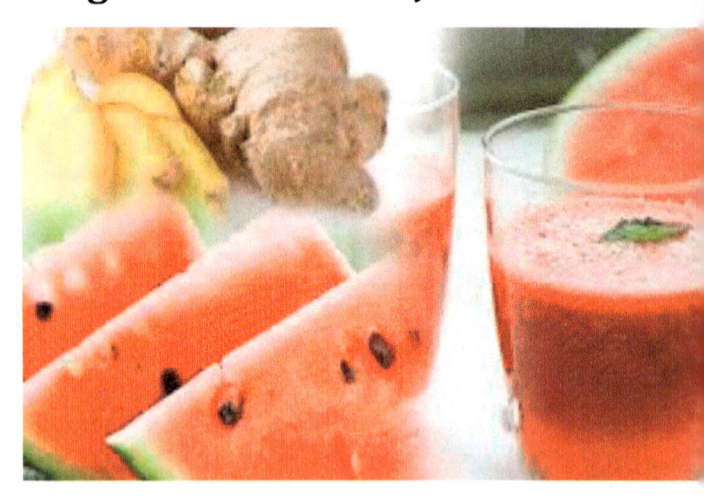

Preparation Time: 15 minutes

Servings: 4

Ingredients:

2 cups fresh watermelon

1 cup frozen strawberries

½ fresh lime

¼ teaspoon ginger

Directions:

Add all the ingredients to the juicer and juice.

The Go-To Juice

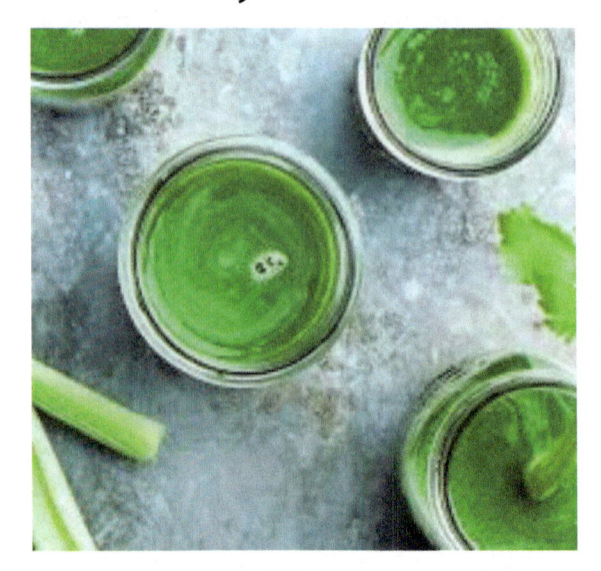

Preparation Time: 10 minutes

Servings: 3

Ingredients:

3 apples

2 carrots

2 celery stalks

4 kale leaves

½ cucumber

Directions:

Start by juicing apples and carrots first, followed by the celery, cucumber then the kale leaves. Serve immediately or refrigerate. The juice will stay good in the refrigerator for up to 24 hours.

Blue Grape-fruity Juice

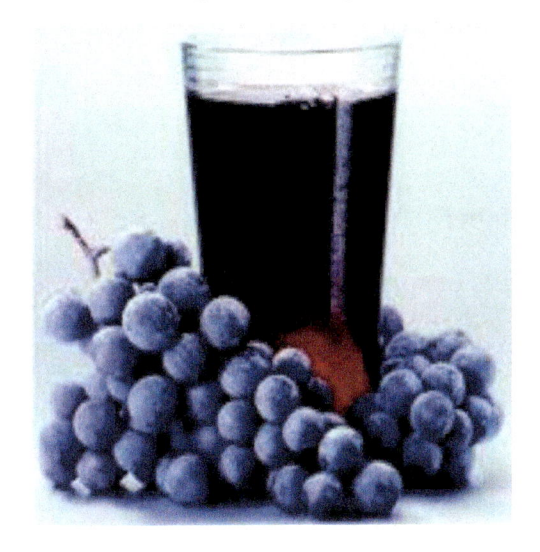

Preparation Time: 15 minutes

Servings: 3

Ingredients:

1/2 of a grapefruit

15 grapes

1 ½ cup of blueberries

½ cup sparkling water

Directions:

Juice all ingredients. Serve immediately or refrigerate. The juice will stay good in the refrigerator for up to 24 hours.

The Belly Settler Juice

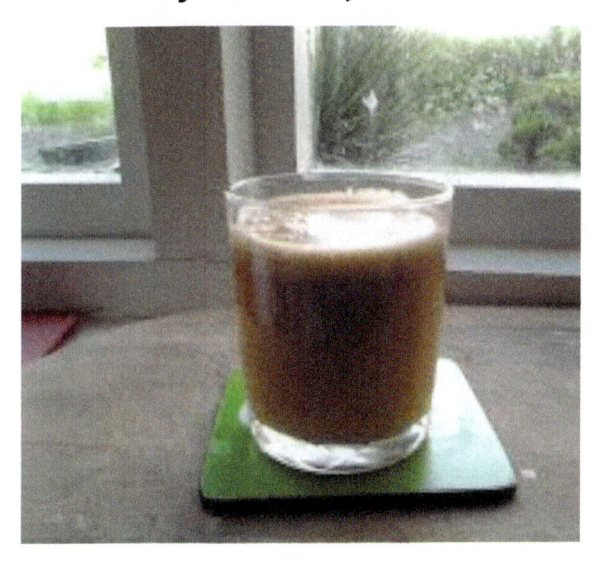

Preparation Time: 10 minutes

Servings: 3

Ingredients:

5 unpeeled carrots

2 apples, cored and cut

12 spinach leaves

1 inch of ginger

Directions:

Juice carrots and apples first, then add spinach and ginger. Serve immediately or refrigerate. The juice will stay good in the refrigerator for up to 24 hours.

Beet Cool Dude Juice

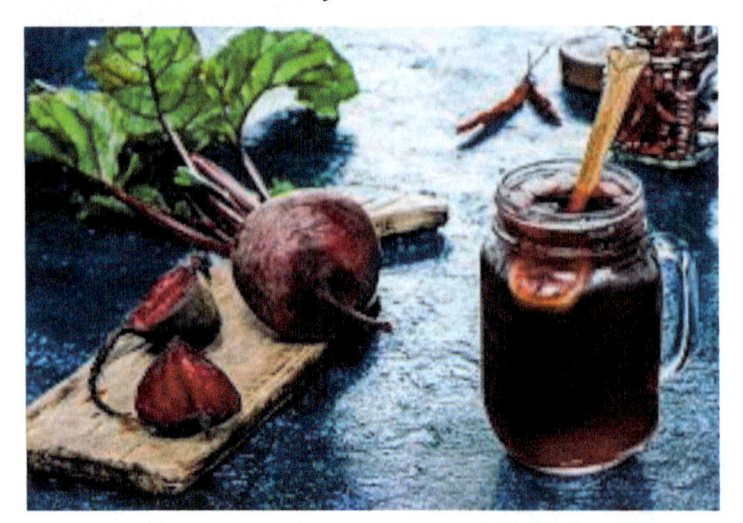

Preparation Time: 15 minutes

Servings: 3

Ingredients:

1/2 of a beet

1/2 of a cucumber

5 Carrots

4 oz. of wheatgrass

Directions:

Juice carrots and cucumber followed by beet and then add wheatgrass. Serve immediately or refrigerate. The juice will stay good in the refrigerator for up to 24 hours.

Green Garlic Monster Juice

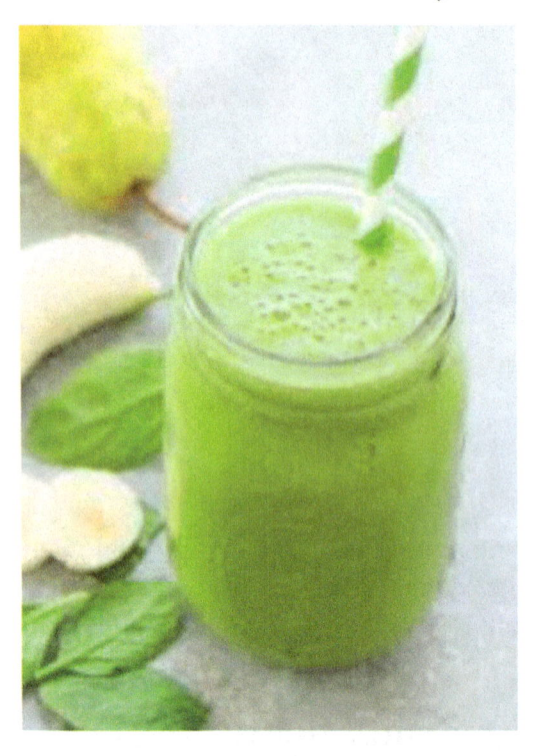

Preparation Time: 10 minutes

Servings: 3

Ingredients:

1/2 of a cucumber

2 large handfuls of spinach

½ cup of cabbage

3 carrots

1 garlic clove

Directions:

Combine all ingredients in the juicer. Serve immediately or refrigerate. The juice will stay good in the refrigerator for up to 24 hours.

Cucumber Beet Juice

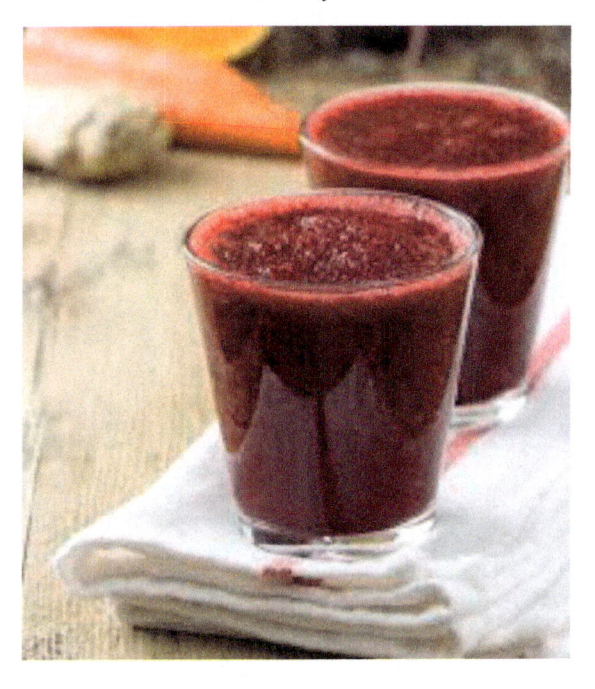

Preparation Time: 15 minutes

Servings: 3

Ingredients:

1 cucumber

3 carrots

1 beet

2 stalks of celery

1 handful of parsley

Half a peeled lemon

Directions:

Juice all ingredients. Serve immediately or refrigerate. The juice will stay good in the refrigerator for up to 24 hours.

Dessert Juice

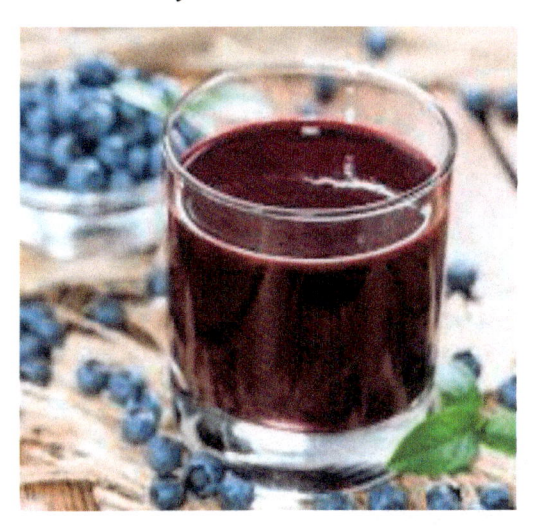

Preparation Time: 10 minutes

Servings: 3

Ingredients:

½ cup of pineapple

½ cup of blueberries

1 Cored apple

Directions:

Juice all ingredients. Serve immediately or refrigerate. The juice will stay good in the refrigerator for up to 24 hours.

Peach Sunrise Juice

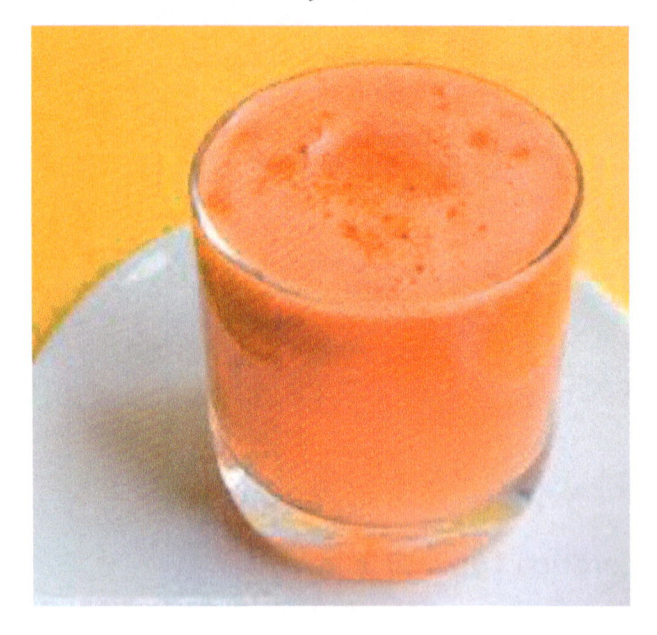

Preparation Time: 15 minutes

Servings: 3

Ingredients:

1 Cup of sliced peaches

½ cup of strawberries

¼ cup of pineapple

1 Peeled orange or 1/2 cup of fresh orange juice

½ cup sparkling water (optional)

Directions:

Juice and combine all ingredients. Serve immediately or refrigerate. The juice will stay good in the refrigerator for up to 24 hours.

Swiss Chard and Goji Berry Juice

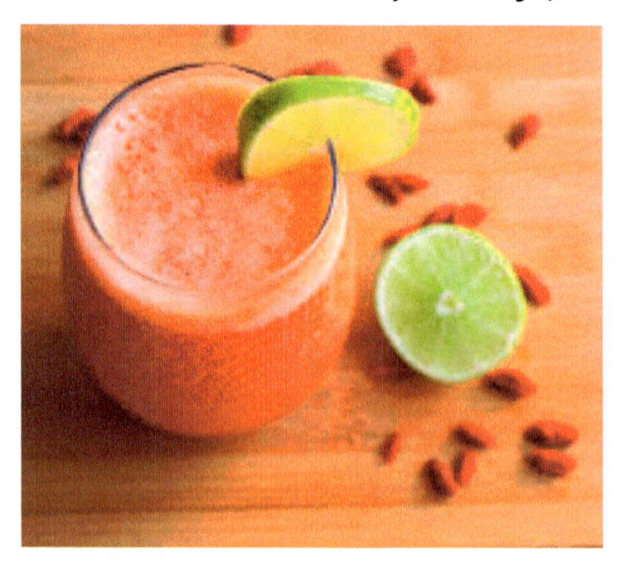

Preparation Time: 15 minutes

Servings: 4

Ingredients:

1 cup swiss Chard

½ cup pineapple

½ cup strawberries

1 tablespoon goji berries

10 cashews

1 ½ cups water

2 ½ teaspoons superfood beauty boost

Directions:

Add all the ingredients to the juicer and juice.

Glowing Skin Juice

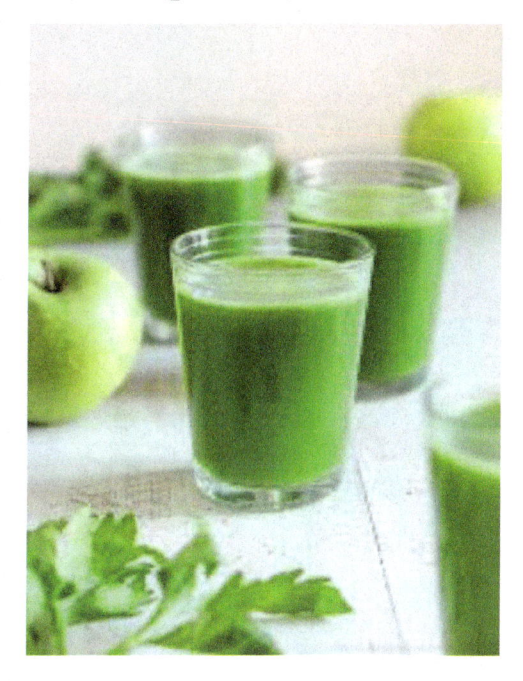

Preparation Time: 15 minutes

Servings: 4

Ingredients:

1 cup swiss Chard

2 tablespoons oats

1 tablespoon cacao

½ cup pineapple

½ cup strawberries

2 tablespoons goji berries

1 ½ cups water

1 teaspoon superfood beauty boost

Directions:

Add all the ingredients to the juicer and juice.

Green Machine Juice

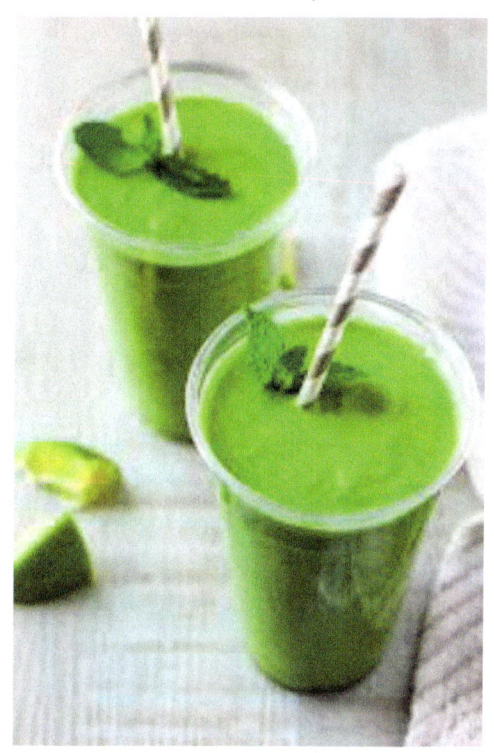

Preparation Time: 10 minutes

Servings: 3

Ingredients:

4 kale leaves

2 apples, cored and cut

2 cups of spinach

½ a cucumber

2 celery sticks

1 medium-sized carrot

1 inch of ginger

Directions:

Combine all ingredients in the juicer. Serve immediately and enjoy or refrigerate. The juice will stay good in the refrigerator for up to 24 hours.

Parsley Energy Juice

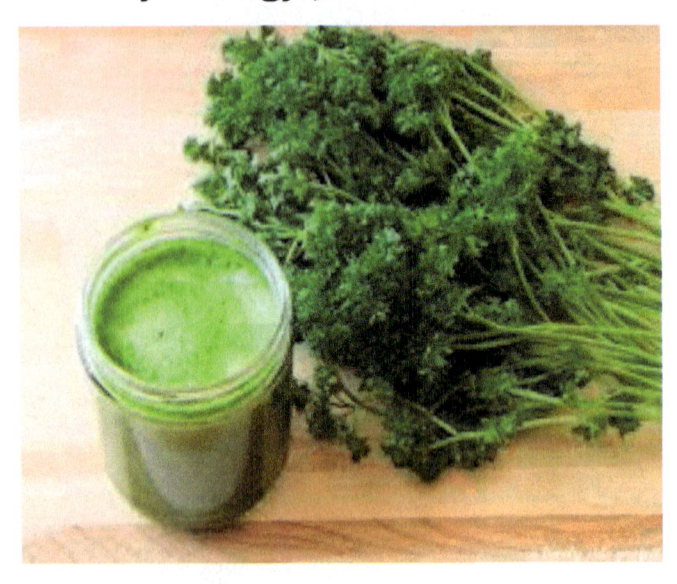

Preparation Time: 10 minutes

Servings: 3

Ingredients:

1 large bunch of parsley

2 carrots

1 apple

1 celery

Directions:

Combine all ingredients in the juicer. Serve immediately and enjoy or refrigerate. The juice will stay good in the refrigerator for up to 24 hours.

Swiss Chard Kale Juice

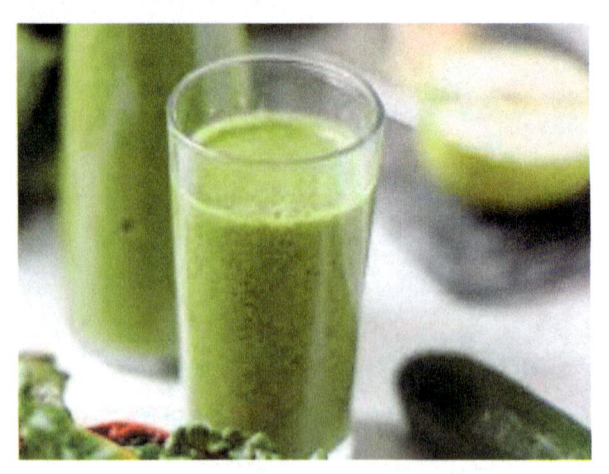

Preparation Time: 10 minutes

Servings: 3

Ingredients:

2 cups of Swiss chard

1 cup of kale

2 medium-sized carrots

2 stalks of celery

2 apples, cored and cut

Directions:

Juice apples, celery, and carrots, then juice kale and chard. Serve immediately or refrigerate. The juice will stay good in the refrigerator for up to 24 hours.

Kiwi Orange Juice

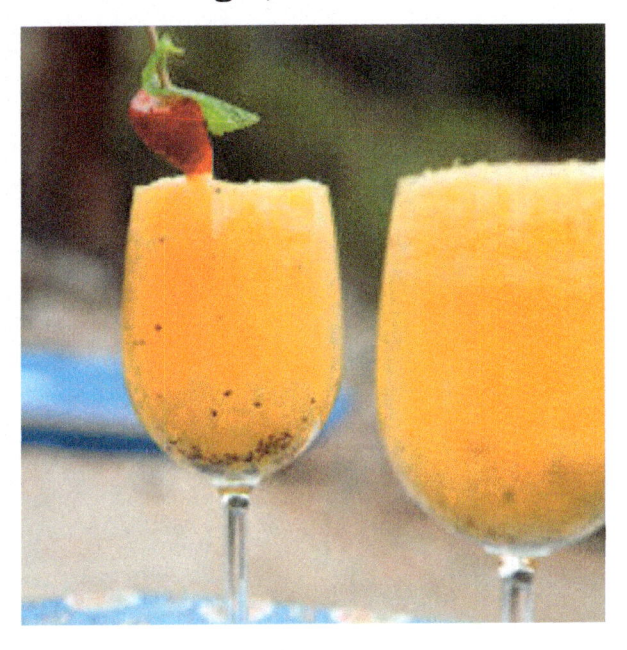

Preparation Time: 10 minutes

Servings: 3

Ingredients:

3 kiwifruits

2 oranges

Freshly squeezed juice from one lemon

1 tangerine

Directions:

Peel orange juice with all ingredients. Serve immediately or refrigerate. The juice will stay good in the refrigerator for up to 24 hours.

Grape-Beet Juice

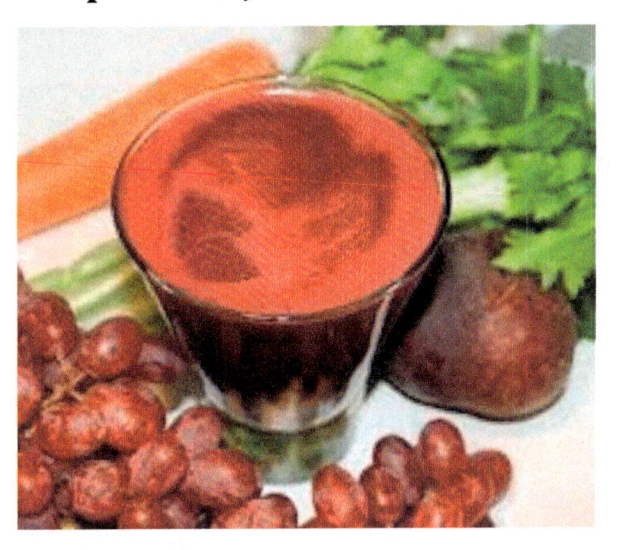

Preparation Time: 15 minutes

Servings: 4

Ingredients:

2 cups red grapes

4 celery stalks

4 beets (peeled)

4 carrots

Directions:

Add all the ingredients to the juicer and juice.

Sweet Potato, Bell Pepper, Beet and Carrot Juice

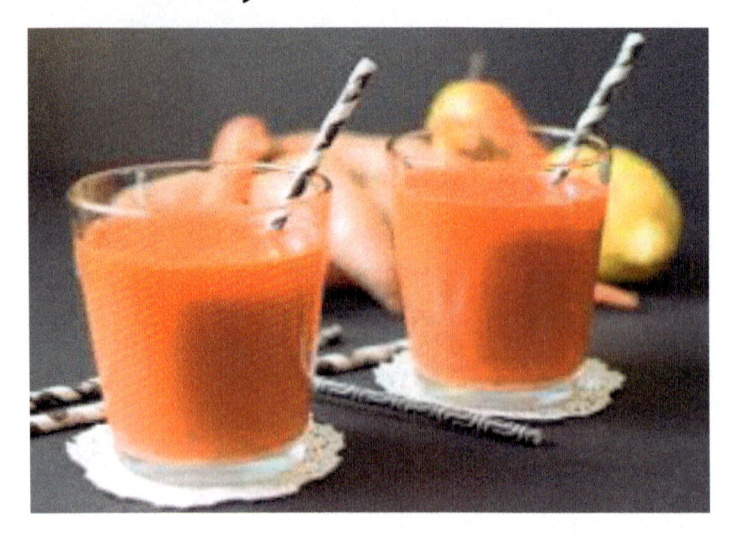

Preparation Time: 10 minutes

Servings: 3

Ingredients:

2 red apples, core removed

2 beets, sliced into wedges

1 cup of sweet potatoes, cut into cubes

1 red bell pepper, seeds removed and thinly sliced

1 carrot, peeled and thinly sliced

Directions:

Wash the red apples, beet, sweet potatoes, red bell pepper, and carrots thoroughly.

In a blender, add in the apples, beet wedges, sweet potato cubes, sliced red bell pepper, and sliced carrots.

Blend on the highest setting until smooth in consistency. Pour into a chilled glass and serve immediately.

Asparagus, Coriander, and Onion Juice

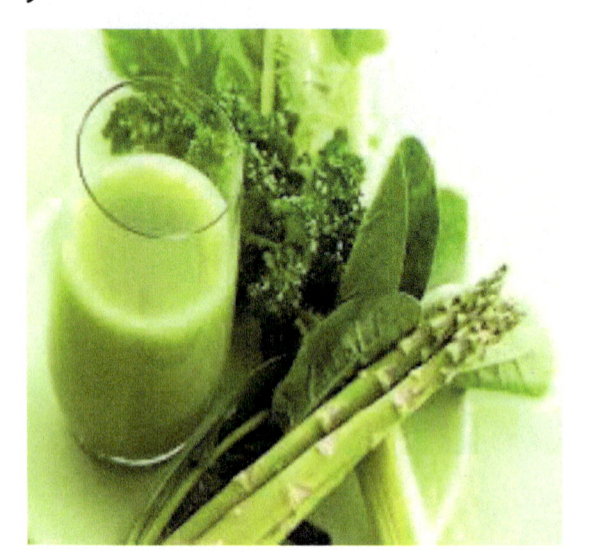

Preparation Time: 10 minutes

Servings: 3

Ingredients:

1/3 cup of asparagus

½ cup of coriander leaves, chopped

1 ½ Tbsp. of white onion, chopped

2 Tbsp. of light brown sugar

1 ½ cup of water, distilled

Directions:

Rinse the asparagus thoroughly. Cut into 1-inch-thick cubes.

Place a saucepan over medium to high heat. Add in 2 cups of water. Add in the asparagus. Boil for 3 to 5 minutes or until bright green. Drain and pat dry.

In a blender, add in the asparagus, chopped coriander leaves, chopped white, light brown sugar, and distilled water.

Blend on the highest setting until smooth in consistency.

Pour into a chilled glass and serve immediately.

Morning Glory Juice

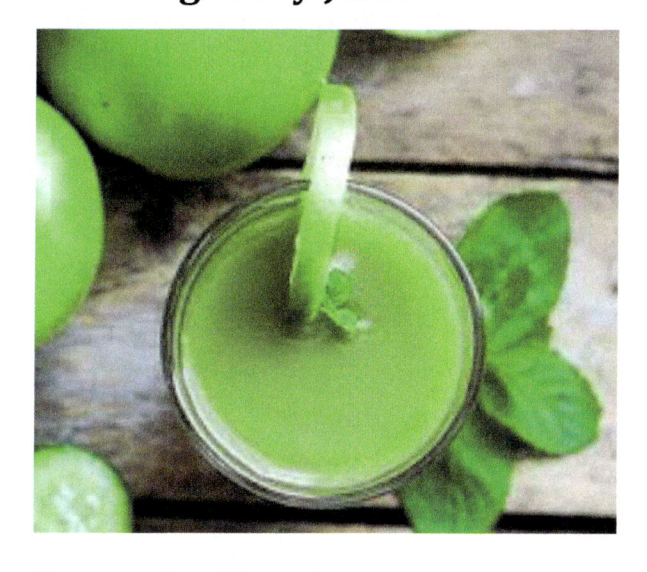

Preparation Time: 20 minutes

Servings: 3

Ingredients:

2 apples

1 cucumber

1 cup of blueberries

2 cups of grapes

2 kale leaves

1 inch of ginger

Directions:

Juice apple and cucumber first, then add grapes and blueberries followed by kale leaves and ginger. Serve immediately and enjoy or refrigerate. The juice will stay good in the refrigerator for up to 24 hours.

Kale Anti-Aging Juice

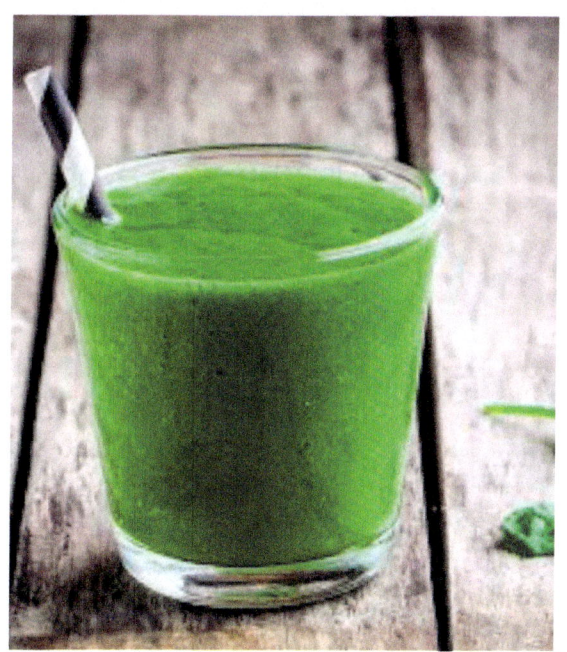

Preparation Time: 15 minutes

Servings: 4

Ingredients:

3 leaves of kale

2 slices of watermelon

2 Apples (seeded)

¼ Lemon (peeled)

Directions:

Add all the ingredients to the juicer and juice.

Mango and Pineapple Juice

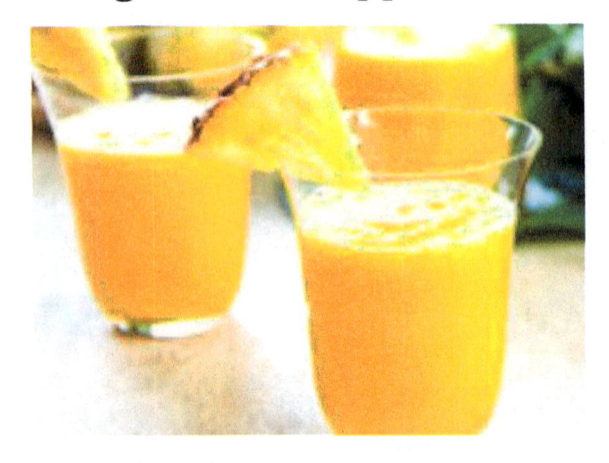

Preparation Time: 15 minutes

Servings: 4

Ingredients:

1 mango (peeled)

1 pineapple (peeled)

Directions:

Add all the ingredients to the juicer and juice.

Broccoli and Pear Juice

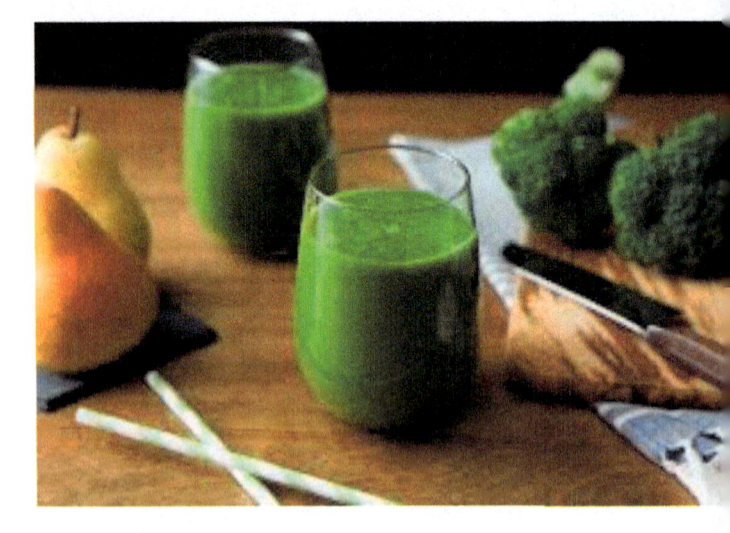

Preparation Time: 15 minutes

Servings: 4

Ingredients:

1 cup broccoli florets

1 ¼ cups pear (cubed)

1 ¼ cups apple (cubed)

¾ cup water

½ teaspoon black salt

½ cup crushed ice

Directions:

Add all the ingredients to the juicer and juice.

Carrot and Pineapple Juice

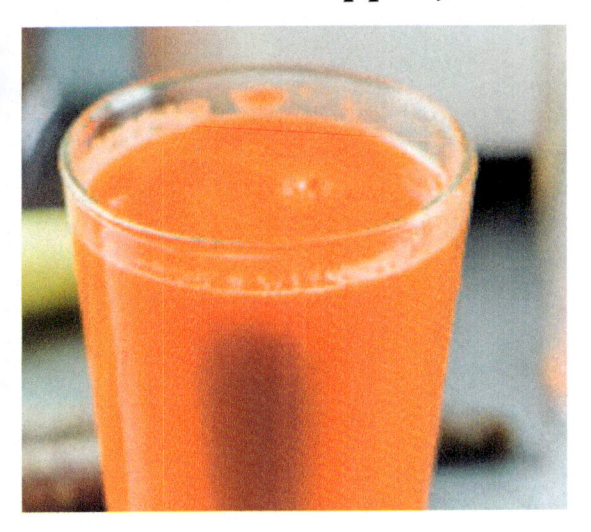

Preparation Time: 15 minutes

Servings: 4

Ingredients:

1/3 pineapple (peeled)

1 orange (peeled)

2 carrots (tailed and topped)

½ lime (peeled)

Directions:

Add all the ingredients to the juicer and juice.

Chapter 7: Juices for Weight Loss

Fresh Cilantro Lettuce Orange juice

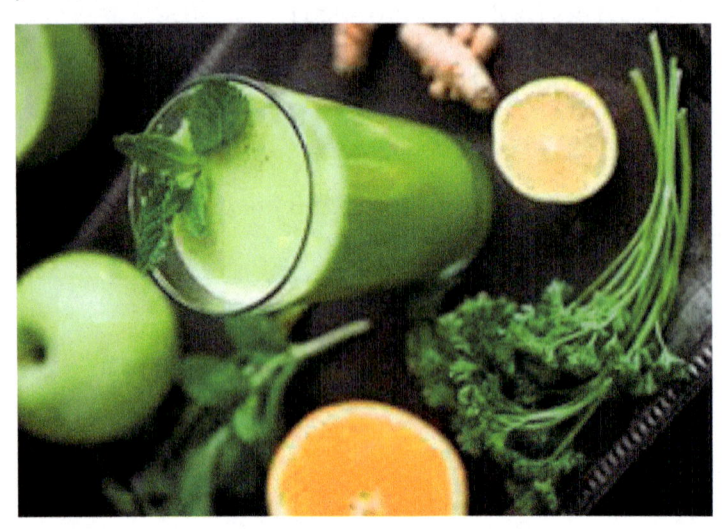

Preparation Time: 10 minutes

Servings: 4

Ingredients:

2 oranges

1 handful fresh cilantro

1 head romaine lettuce

2 kale leaves

2 celery stalks

Directions:

Add all ingredients into the juicer and blend.

Serve and enjoy.

Broccoli Mint Apple Juice

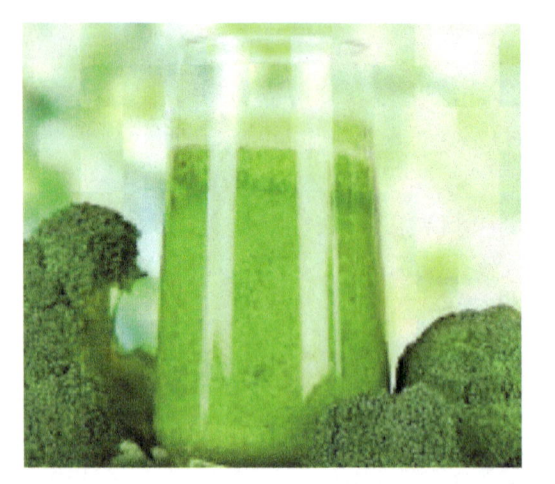

Preparation Time: 15 minutes

Servings: 4

Ingredients:

1 handful fresh mint

1/2 fresh lemon

1 cucumber

1 whole broccoli

1 apple

Directions:

Add all ingredients into the juicer and blend.

Serve and enjoy.

Grapefruit Mint Lettuce Juice

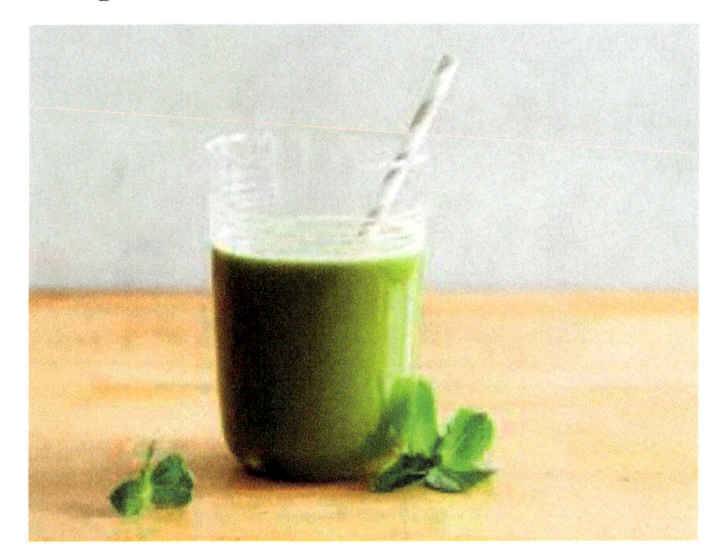

Preparation Time: 15 minutes

Servings: 4

Ingredients:

1 head romaine lettuce

1 bunch mint leaves

2 oranges, peeled

1 grapefruit, peeled

Directions:

Add all ingredients into the juicer and blend.

Serve and enjoy.

Grape Spinach Kiwi Juice

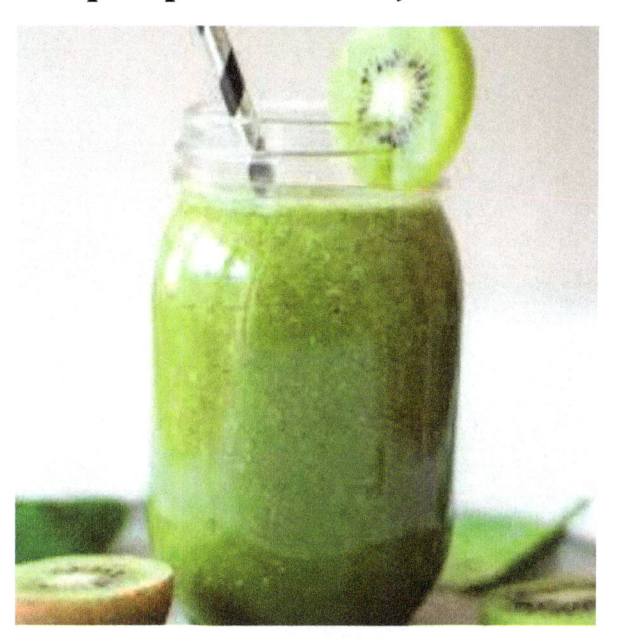

Preparation Time: 15 minutes

Servings: 4

Ingredients:

2 cups cold water

2 kiwis

1/2 cup fresh spinach

1 cup green grapes

1/2 cucumber

Directions:

Add all ingredients into the juicer and blend.

Serve and enjoy.

Kale Powerade Juice

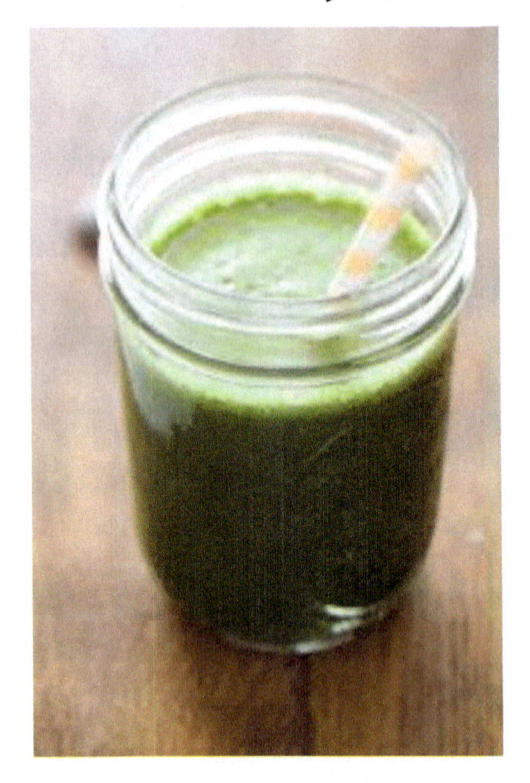

Preparation Time: 10 minutes

Servings: 4

Ingredients:

1 cup kale
¾ cup spinach
1 carrot
½ beet, with leaves
1 apple

Directions:

Chop vegetables and apple into chunks. Feed soft and hard ingredients alternatively to juice. Kale is packed full of protein, vitamins, and nutrients.

Mexican Bell Pepper Juice

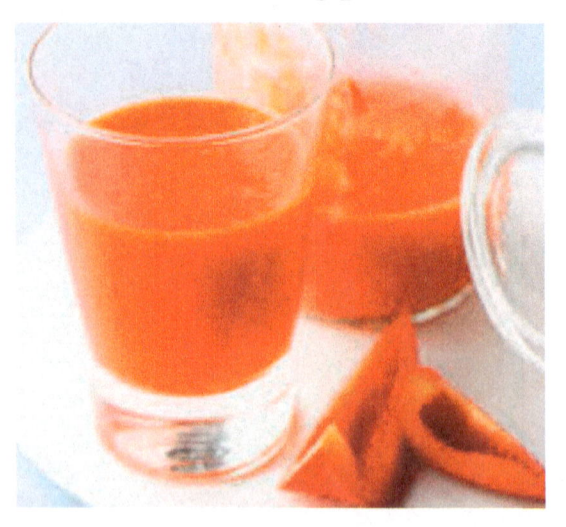

Preparation Time: 10 minutes

Servings: 4

Ingredients:

2 apples

1/2 bell pepper

2 cucumbers

1 bunch of cilantro

½ lime

Directions:

Add all the ingredients to the juicer and juice.

Refreshing Apple Mint Juice

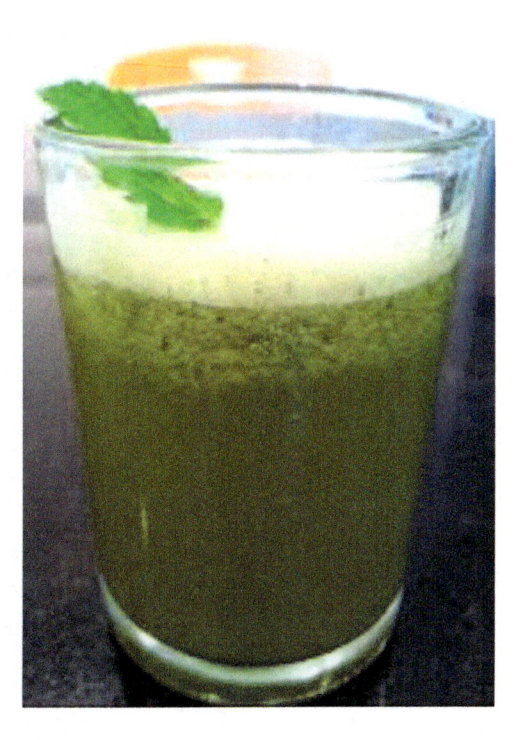

Preparation Time: 10 minutes

Servings: 4

Ingredients:

1 cucumber

1 orange

1 lemon

1/2 lb. fresh mint leaves

1/2 lb. green apples

Directions:

Add all ingredients into the juicer and blend. Serve and enjoy.

Dandelion Parsley Kale Juice

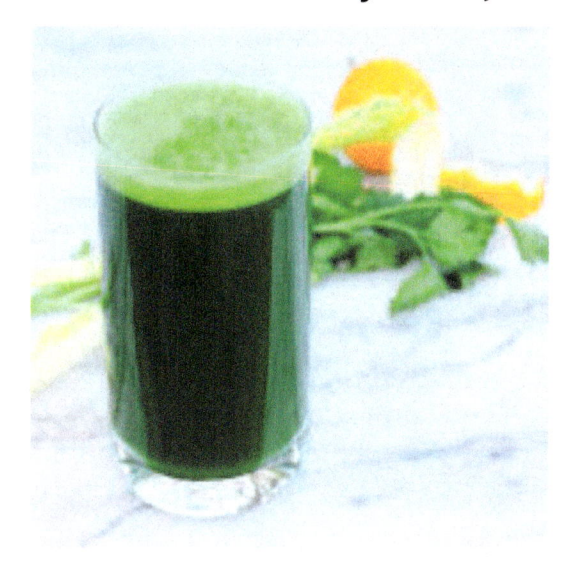

Preparation Time: 10 minutes

Servings: 4

Ingredients:

1/2 lb. celery

1 lb. cucumber

1/4 lb. fresh parsley

1/2 lb. kale leaves

1/2 lb. dandelion greens

Directions:

Add all ingredients into the juicer and blend.

Serve and enjoy.

Spinach Ginger Lemon Juice

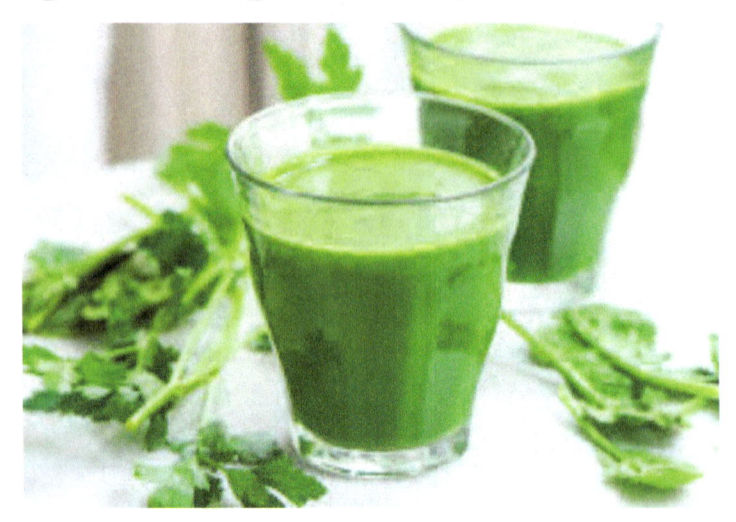

Preparation Time: 10 minutes

Servings: 4

Ingredients:

1 cup fresh spinach

1-inch fresh ginger

2 lemons

1 tbsp maple syrup

Directions :

Add all ingredients into the juicer and blend.

Serve and enjoy.

Protein: 6.3g

Sugars: 6.6g

Mint Watercress Beet Juice

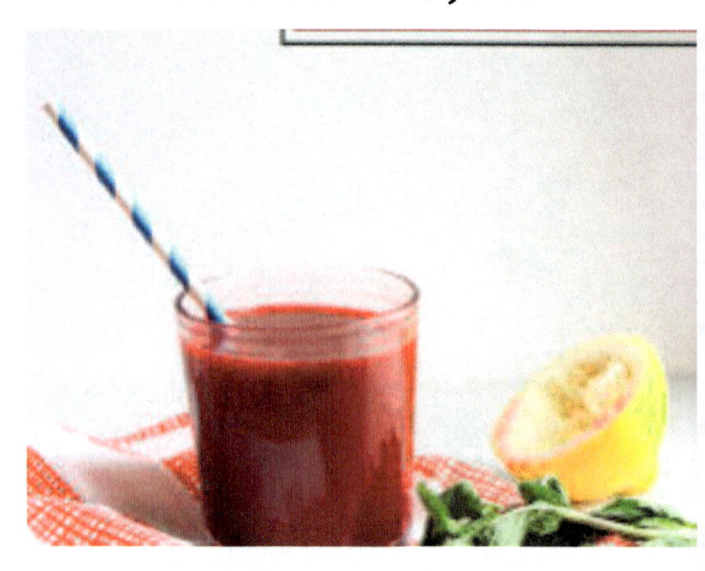

Preparation Time: 10 minutes

Servings: 4

Ingredients:

3 tbsp fresh mint leaves

1/2 daikon radish

1 bunch of watercress leaves

1 beet

2 carrots

Directions:

Add all ingredients into the juicer and blend.

Serve and enjoy.

Kiwi and Cucumber Juice

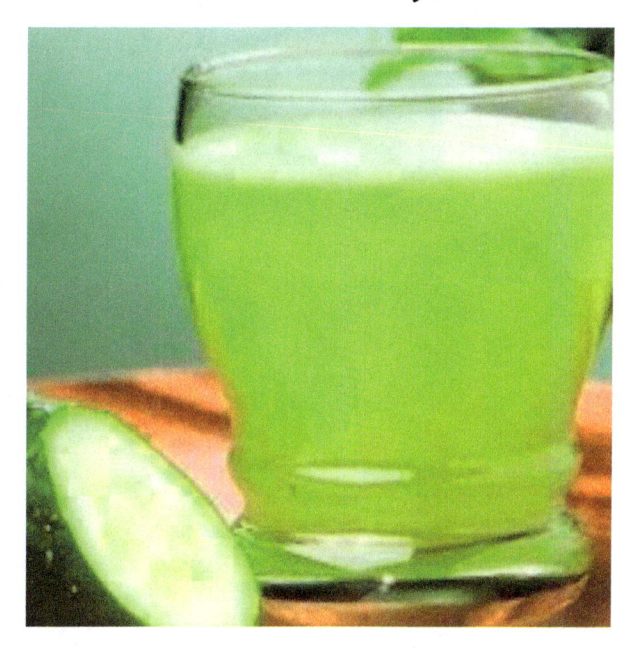

Preparation Time: 15 minutes

Servings: 4

Ingredients:

1 cucumber

1 apple

1 kiwi (only flesh)

Directions:

Add all the ingredients to the juicer and juice.

Carrot and Broccoli Juice

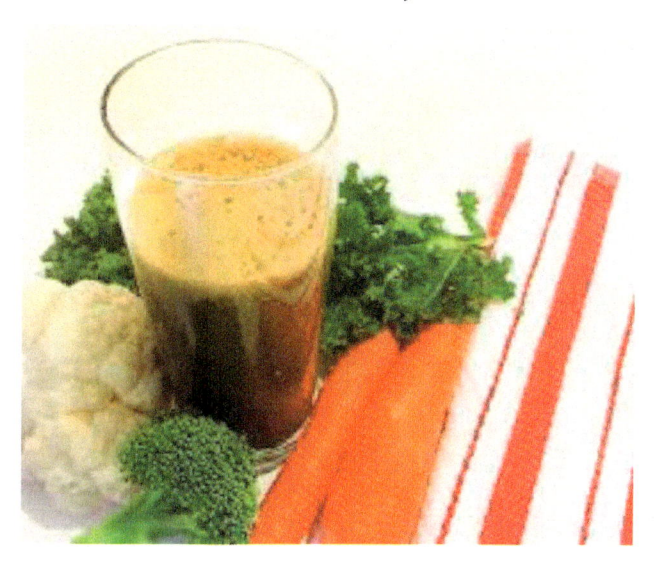

Preparation Time: 15 minutes

Servings: 4

Ingredients:

¼ cucumber

2 carrots

1 potato

2 broccoli florets

½ beet

¼ red bell pepper

1 tomato

Directions:

Add all the ingredients to the juicer and juice.

Ginger Garlic Green Juice

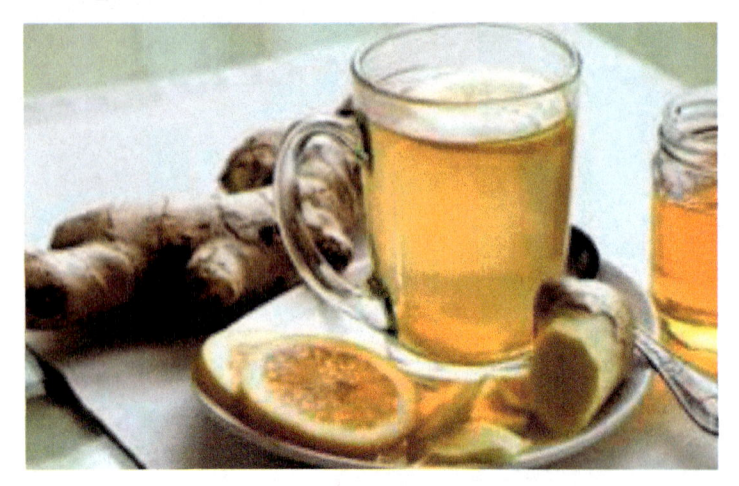

Preparation Time: 15 minutes

Servings: 4

Ingredients:

1-inch fresh ginger

1 garlic clove

1 green apple

4 carrots, peeled

1 handful parsley

1 handful fresh spinach

Directions:

Add all ingredients into the juicer and blend.

Serve and enjoy.

Green Juice for Healthy Eye

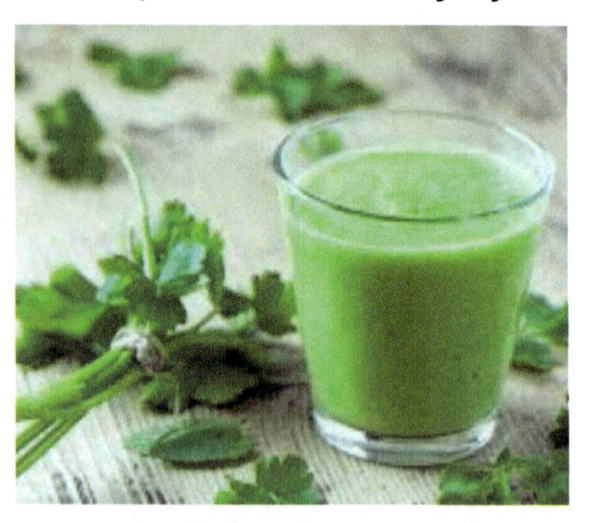

Preparation Time: 15 minutes

Servings: 4

Ingredients:

1 fresh lime

2 handful kale

3 handful fresh cilantro

1 cucumber

4 medium carrots

Directions:

Add all ingredients into the juicer and blend.

Serve and enjoy.

Melon and Wheatgrass Juice

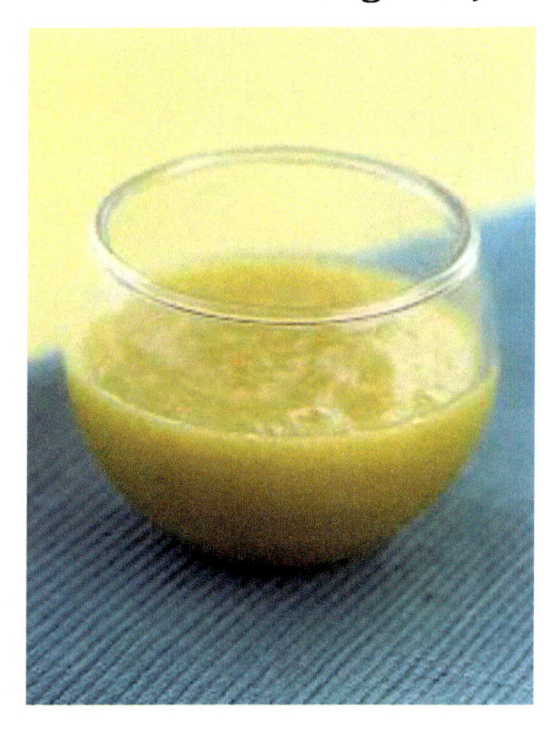

Preparation Time: 15 minutes

Servings: 4

Ingredients:

1 ½ cups muskmelon (deseeded, cubed)

1 cup watermelon (cubed)

2 tablespoons wheatgrass (chopped)

8 orange segments

Directions:

Add all the ingredients to the juicer and juice.

Watercress and Apple Juice

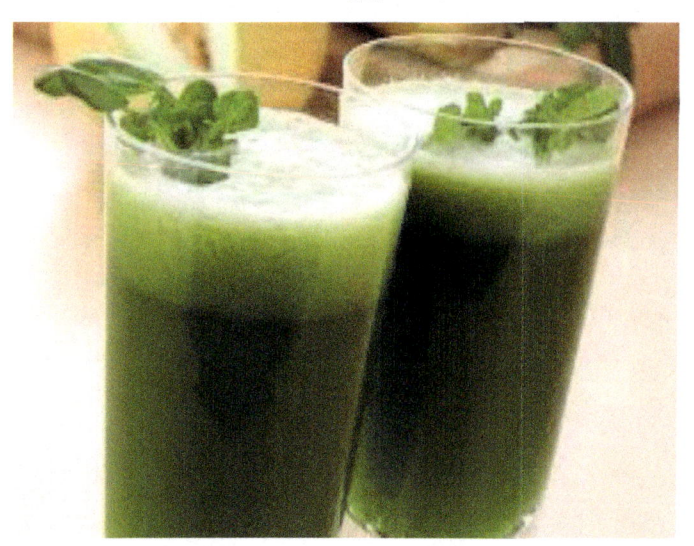

Preparation Time: 15 minutes

Servings: 4

Ingredients:

2 apples

1 cup blackberries

4 ¾ oz watercress

Directions:

Add all the ingredients to the juicer and juice.

Lemony Grapefruit Juice

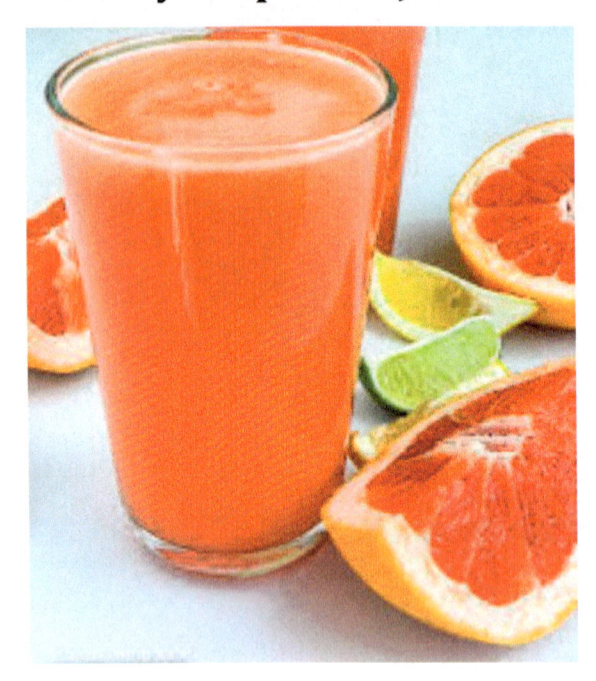

Preparation Time: 15 minutes

Servings: 4

Ingredients:

1 bitter melon

½ grapefruit

1 lemon (unpeeled)

Directions:

Add all the ingredients to the juicer and juice.

Citrus Mango Juice

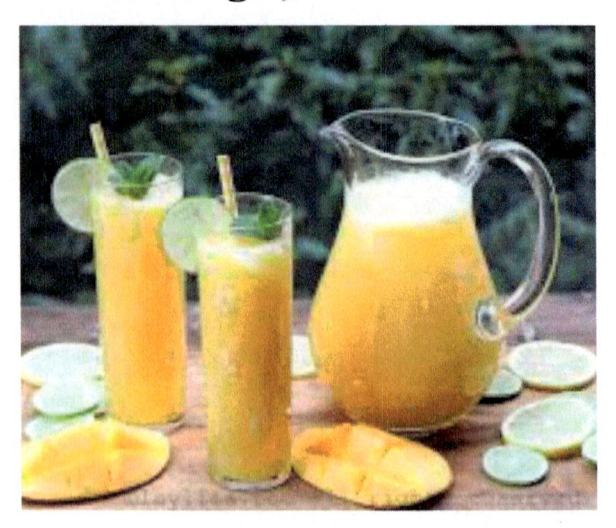

Preparation Time: 15 minutes

Servings: 4

Ingredients:

1 mango

Lime juice of 1 lime

½ cup water

Directions:

Add all the ingredients to the juicer and juice.

Simple Nice Green Juice

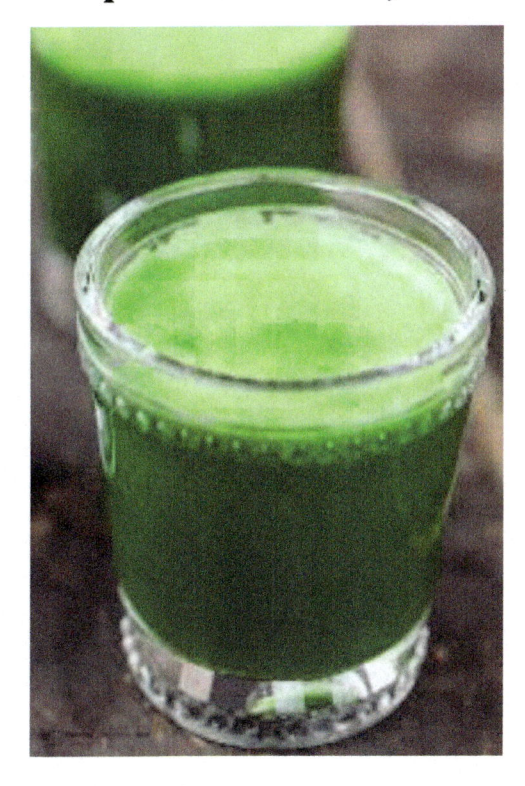

Preparation Time: 15 minutes

Servings: 4

Ingredients

2 large apples of 3-inch diameter

8 large celery stalks of 11-inch length

1 lemon fruit with peel

1 peeled orange fruit

Directions:

Add the ingredients to your juice

Juice them thoroughly until you have a smooth juice

Pour the drink into a glass and give it a nice shakeChill and serve!

"Kitchen Sink" Detox Juice

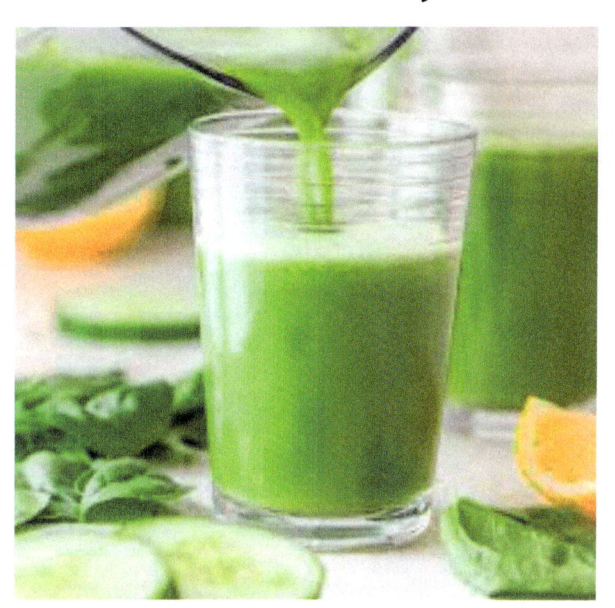

Preparation Time: 20 minutes

Servings: 4

Ingredients:

1/2 cup baby spinach
2 small carrots, chopped
2 apples, chopped
2 sticks celery, chopped
1 tomato
1/4 cucumber, chopped
1 cup strawberries
1 kiwi fruit
1/4 lemon
1/2-inch piece of ginger
1/2 cup kale

Directions:

Bunch up the leafy greens and feed them through the juicer machine alternating with the other ingredients. This really is a super healthy detox juice packed full of a home-grown garden patch! *Almost* everything, including the kitchen sink!

Crazy Cabbage Juice

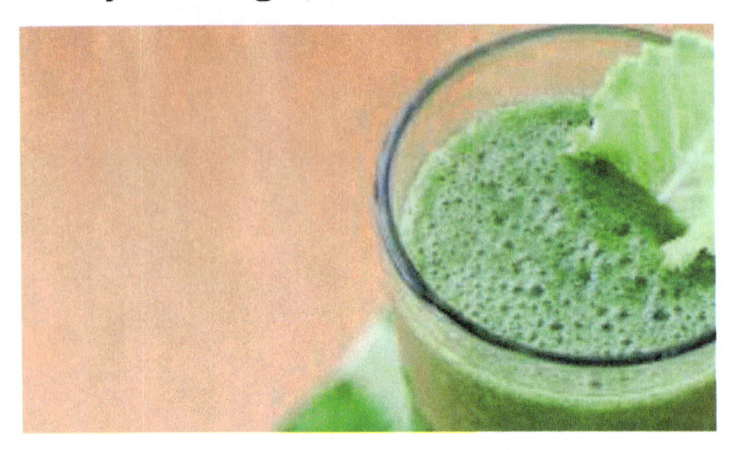

Preparation Time: 20 minutes

Servings: 4

Ingredients:

1/2 cabbage, chopped with lower stalk removed
2 carrots, chopped
4 celery sticks

Directions:

Juice the cabbage first, then the carrots and celery. Cabbage is good for the stomach and is known to help treat peptic ulcers. The carotene-rich carrots also give a powerful punch. Can add an apple or some grapes for added sweetness.

Citrus Weight Buster Juice

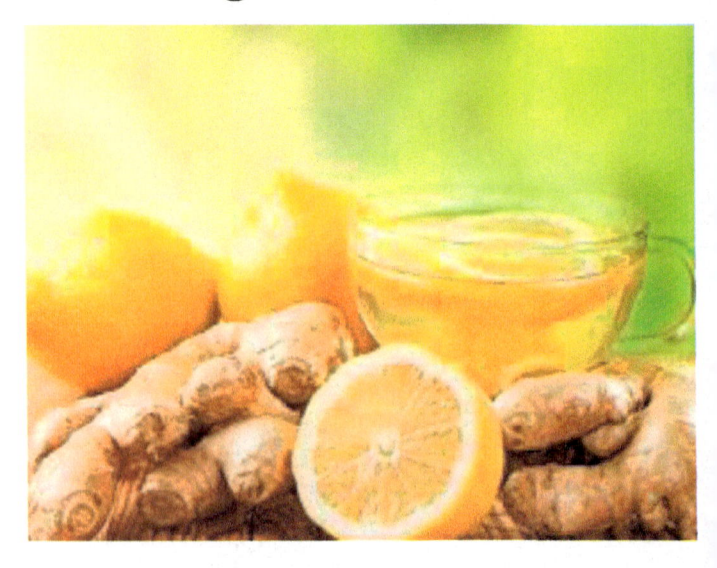

Preparation Time: 10 minutes

Servings: 4

Ingredients:

2 oranges, peeled and quartered
1/2 grapefruit, peeled
1/2 lemon, peeled but keep about a tsp size of peel (optional)
½ lime, peeled

Directions:

Peel fruits but keep 1/4 of the lemon peel on for extra cold-fighting properties. Lemon peels are also full of super-flavonoids helping reduce bad cholesterol. I find this recipe can be hard on the tummy, so eat something with it, or dilute with water. Refreshing summertime weight loss drink and a soother for winter colds!

Sparkling Health Drink Juice

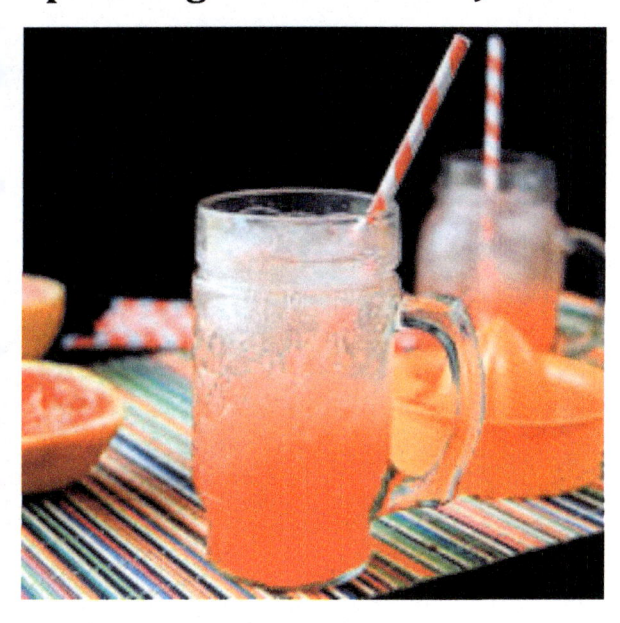

Preparation Time: 10 minutes

Servings: 4

Ingredients:

1 little bunch of parsley or watercress
4 broccoli florets
1/4 pineapple, peeled and chopped
1 in-season sweet apple, chopped (1 /4 cup strawberries work too)
1/4 - 1/2 cup sparkling mineral water
(You can add 1/2 a blended banana for a low GI juice)

Directions:

Bunch up the parsley and feed all ingredients through the juicer alternating together and serve. Mix with sparkling mineral water to taste. A healthy juice full of vitamin C and vital green nutrients, *and* it's yummy! You can change up the juice by leaving out the apple and using 1/2 pineapple. You can also leave out the broccoli and use baby spinach leaves.

Weight Loss Tonic Juice

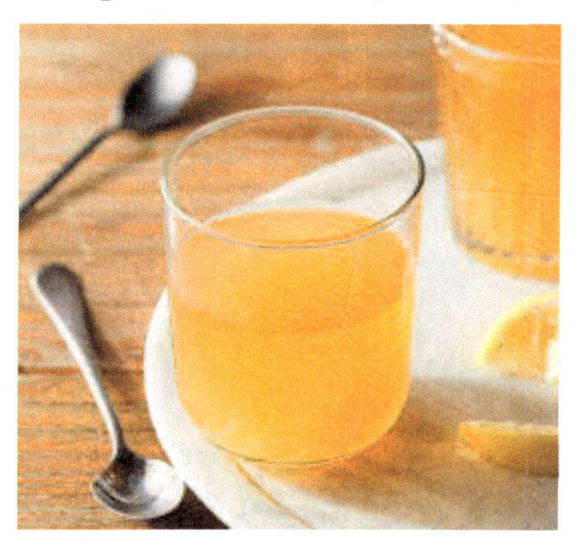

Preparation Time: 10 minutes

Servings: 4

Ingredients:

4 strawberries
4 broccoli florets
1/4 cup alfalfa sprouts
1 apple, chopped
1 sprig parsley
1/2 cup baby spinach leaves
1 orange, peeled, and chopped (leave some of the white on for vitamins)

Directions:

Juice all ingredients, alternating as you go. This is a tasty vitamin-packed favorite in our family. This is an easy, basic juice with the ingredients usually on hand. You can change it up by substituting pineapple or pear for the apple sweet balance, or by using kale or standard spinach instead of baby spinach. Blend in any of the above veggies or fruits in the picture and see if you like it. Great for breakfast, lunch, or a snack.

Apple Cucumber Basil Juice

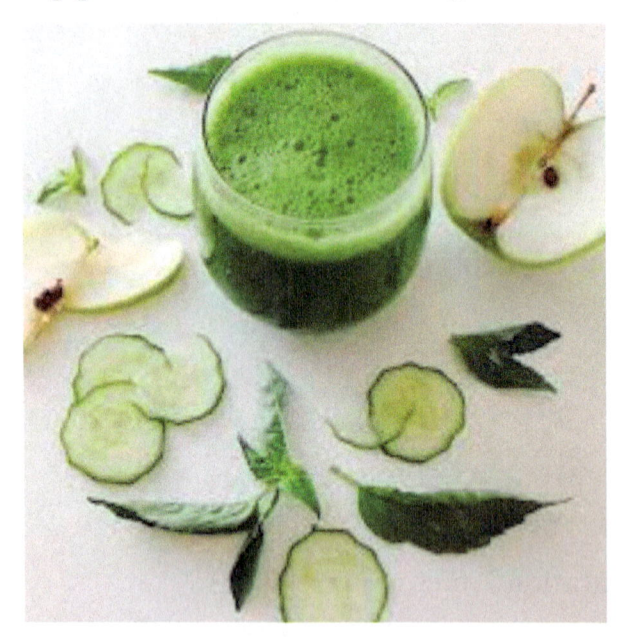

Preparation Time: 10 minutes

Servings: 5

Ingredients:

1 fresh lime

1 medium cucumber

2 green apples

1 handful basil

Directions:

Add all ingredients into the juicer and blend.

Serve and enjoy.

Parsley Lime Pineapple Juice

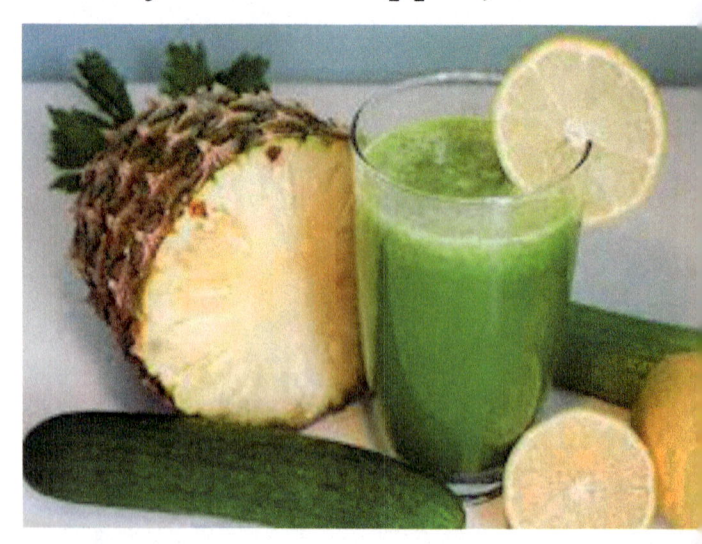

Preparation Time: 10 minutes

Servings: 4

Ingredients:

1 green apple

1/2 cup parsley

1-inch fresh ginger

2 lemons, cut off the skin

1 cup pineapple

1 medium cucumber

Directions:

Add all ingredients into the juicer and blend.

Serve and enjoy.

Apple Pear Swiss chard Juice

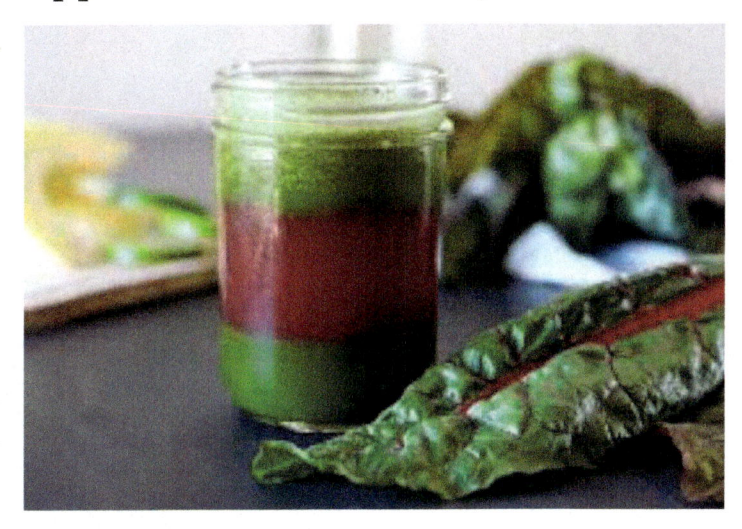

Preparation Time: 10 minutes

Servings: 4

Ingredients:

2 green apples

1 medium cucumber

2 lemons, peeled

1 pear

1 bunch Swiss chard

1 tsp honey

Directions:

Add all ingredients into the juicer and blend. Serve and enjoy.

Coconut Pineapple Lettuce Juice

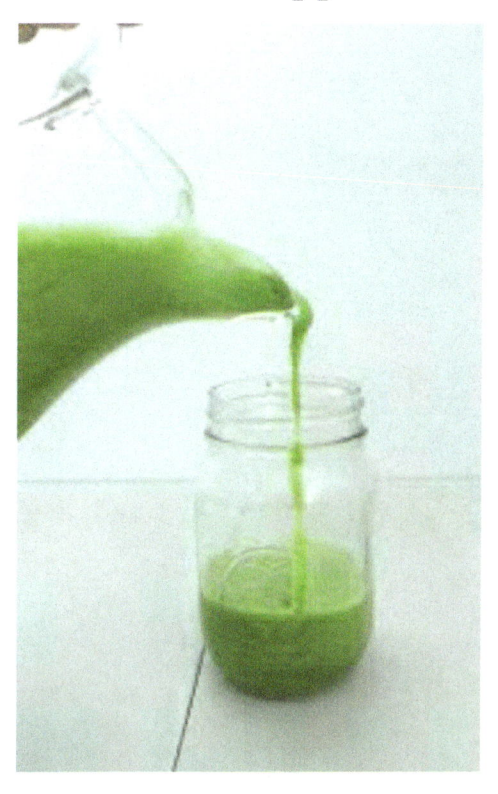

Preparation Time: 15 minutes

Servings: 4

Ingredients:

1/4 cup coconut water

1/2-inch fresh ginger

2 cups pineapple

2 celery stalks

1 heart of romaine lettuce

1/2 cucumber

Directions:

Add all ingredients into the juicer and blend. Serve and enjoy.

Chard Lime Green Juice

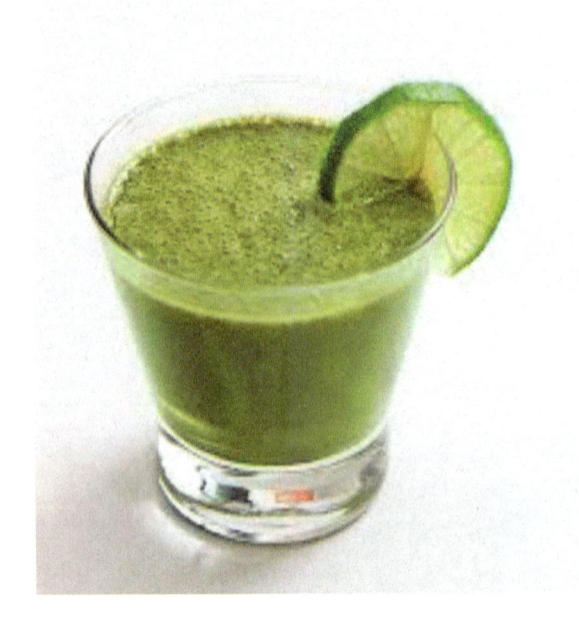

Preparation Time: 15 minutes

Servings: 4

Ingredients:

1 medium apple

1/2 lemon

2 medium cucumbers

4 chard leaves

Directions:

Add all ingredients into the juicer and blend.

Serve and enjoy.

Refreshing Lean Green Juice

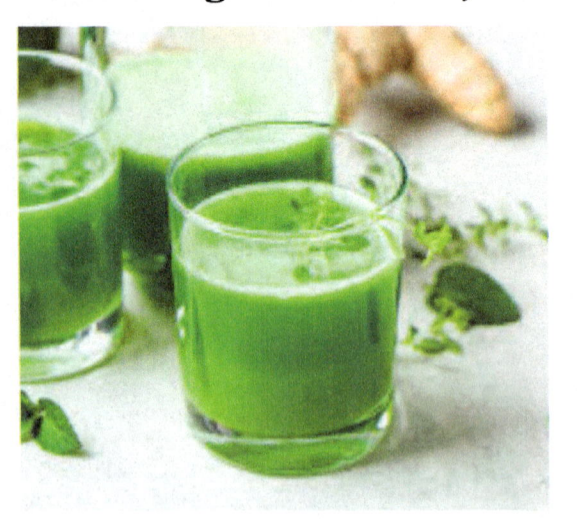

Preparation Time: 15 minutes

Servings: 4

Ingredients:

10 mint leaves

1 cup fresh spinach

1 fresh lime juice

1/2 pear

1/2 cucumber

1/2 cup pineapple

Ice cubes

1 tsp honey

Directions:

Add all ingredients into the juicer and blend.

Serve and enjoy.

Cool as a Cucumber Juice

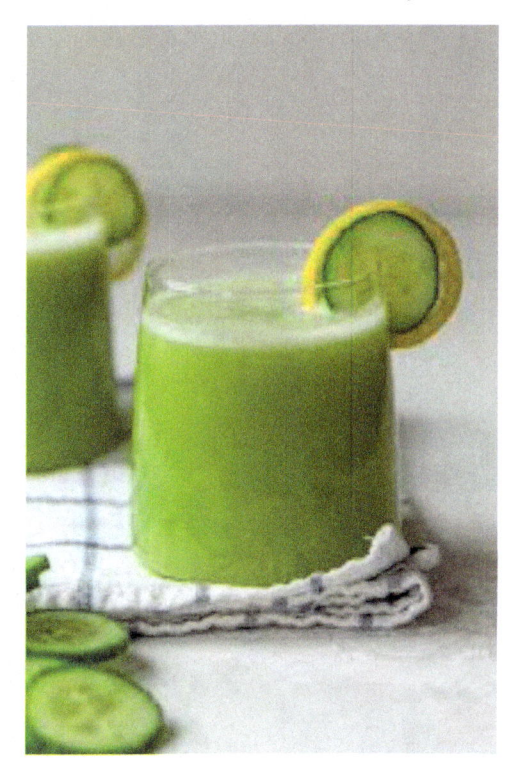

Preparation Time: 15 minutes

Servings: 4

Ingredients:

1 whole cucumber, chopped
1 large green apple, chopped
1 – 2 sticks of celery

Directions:

Simply wash, cut, and core ingredients, place into juicer and juice. For a little twist, add ½ a pomegranate to give it a wonderful sour jolt to enliven your system!

Cinnamon Circulation Booster Juice

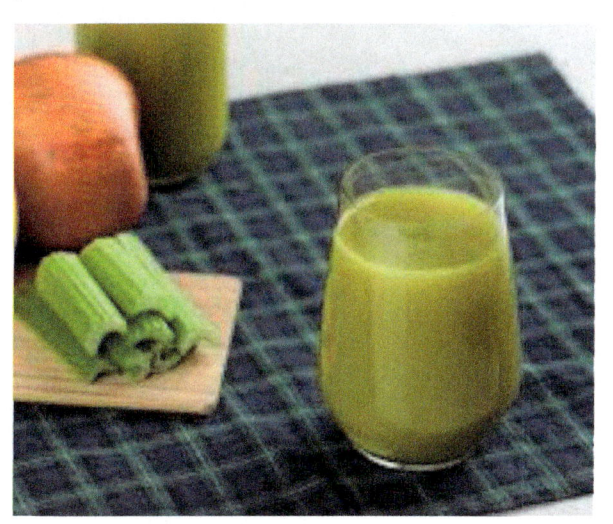

Preparation Time: 20 minutes

Servings: 4

Ingredients:

1/2-inch piece of ginger
1/2 tsp cinnamon
6 small apples, chopped

Directions:

Juice the ginger and apple. Pour into glasses, divide the cinnamon between the two, and stir in. This warming concoction is great before bedtime on a winter's night. The ginger and cinnamon are good for your liver too. Ginger is also known to help improve digestion and circulation.

Antioxidant Bok Choy Juice

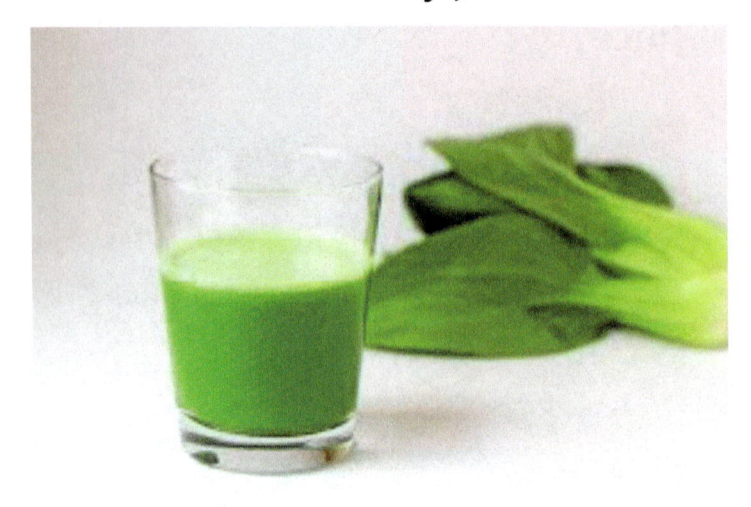

Preparation Time: 20 minutes

Servings: 4

Ingredients:
1 lemon, peeled
1 large or 2 small bok choy (sometimes I add kale or spinach)
1 beet
3 carrots, chopped
3 sticks celery
1 apple, chopped
1/2 cup natural blackcurrant juice, or blackcurrants (optional)

Directions:

Remove and discard the very base from the bok choy. Juice everything leaving the apple till last. Packed full of vitamin C and also great for the skin and liver! Mix up the greens and use whatever you have in the fridge.

Low Cal Tropical Punch Juice

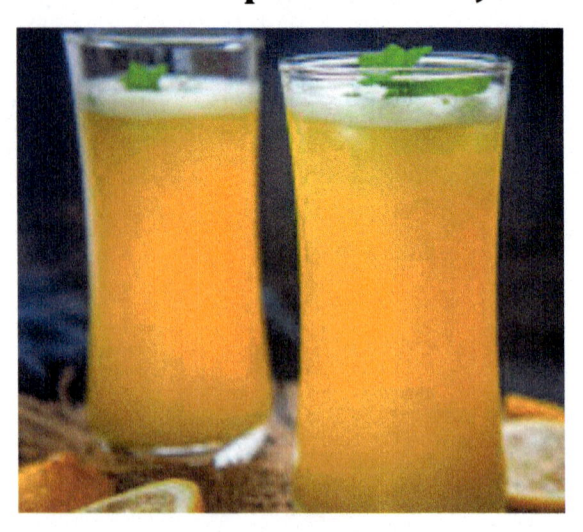

Preparation Time: 20 minutes

Servings: 4

Ingredients:

1 papaya (or mango)
1 large fresh, tinned, or homemade preserved peach
2 passionfruit
150ml orange juice or 1 halved and peeled orange Serve with ice and a shot of vodka or white rum (optional)

Directions:

Remove papaya or mango seed, chop roughly and feed into the juicer. Add stoned and halved peach and orange. Juice, then pour into glasses with ice cubes. Mix in passionfruit pulp including seeds and vodka.

Berry Super Lunch Juice

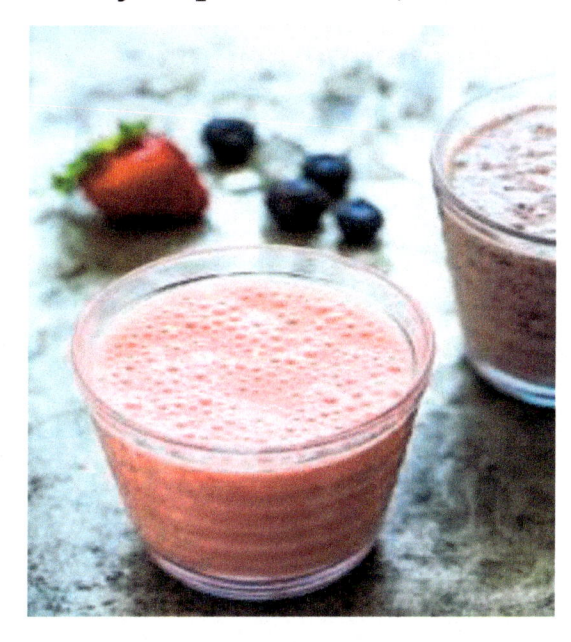

Preparation Time: 20 minutes

Servings: 4

Ingredients:

1 orange, peeled and chopped
2 bananas, peeled and blended on their own first
2 dates
A large handful of Swiss chard or spinach
1 cup blackberries or raspberries (a mix of both is even better)
1 kiwi fruit
1/2 cup strawberries
1 cup water

Directions:

Blend the banana separately. Prepare the orange and push the chard through with this. Then add the other ingredients. Mix with the banana to make a super smoothie drink. This juice is a delicious energy booster and wonderful for a weight watcher's breakfast or lunch!

Hungry Orange Crush Juice

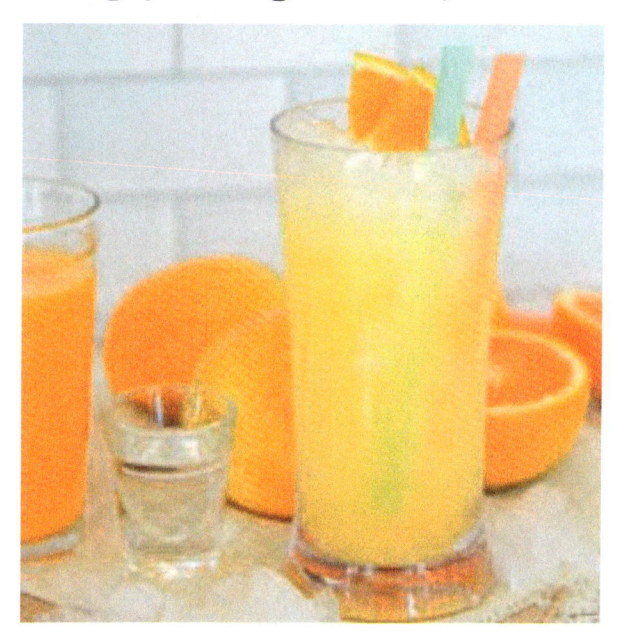

Preparation Time: 10 minutes

Servings: 4

Ingredients

1 medium apple of 3-inch diameter

½ a fruit of lemon of 2-inch diameter

1 large, peeled orange of 3-inch diameter

1 large peach of 2-inch diameter

¼ of a pineapple fruit

Directions:

Add the ingredients to your juicer.

Juice them thoroughly until you have a smooth juice.

Pour the drink into a glass and give it a nice shake.

Chill and serve!

Citrus and Mango Love Juice

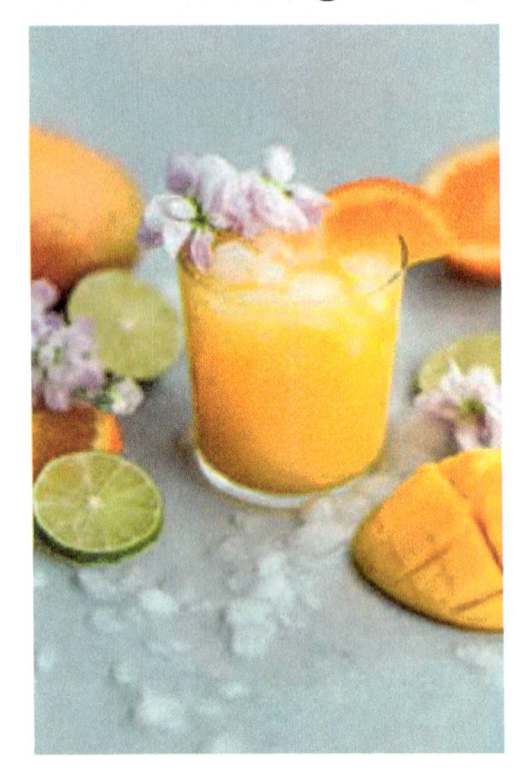

Preparation Time: 10 minutes

Servings: 4

Ingredients

1 large apple of 3-inch diameter

A pinch of cayenne pepper

½ of a lemon fruit peeled up

1 whole mango peeled

1 whole large orange peeled

Directions:

Add the ingredients to your juicer.

Juice them thoroughly until you have a smooth juice.

Pour the drink into a glass and give it a nice shake.

Chill and serve!

Pear Lemon Cucumber Juice

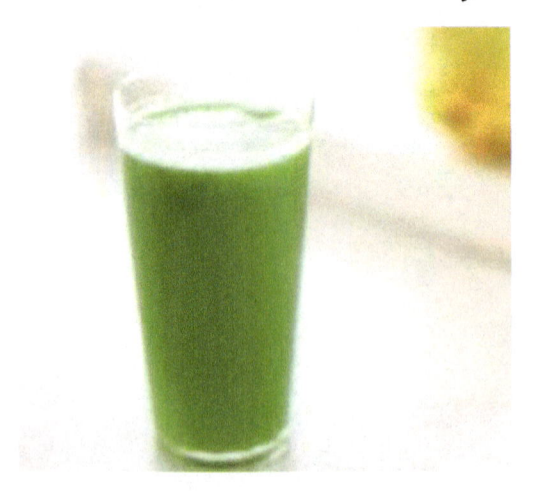

Preparation Time: 15 minutes

Servings: 4

Ingredients:

1 cucumber

1/2 lemon

2 medium pears

2 lettuce heads

Directions:

Add all ingredients into the juicer and blend.

Serve immediately and enjoy.

Watercress Cucumber Blackberry Green Juice

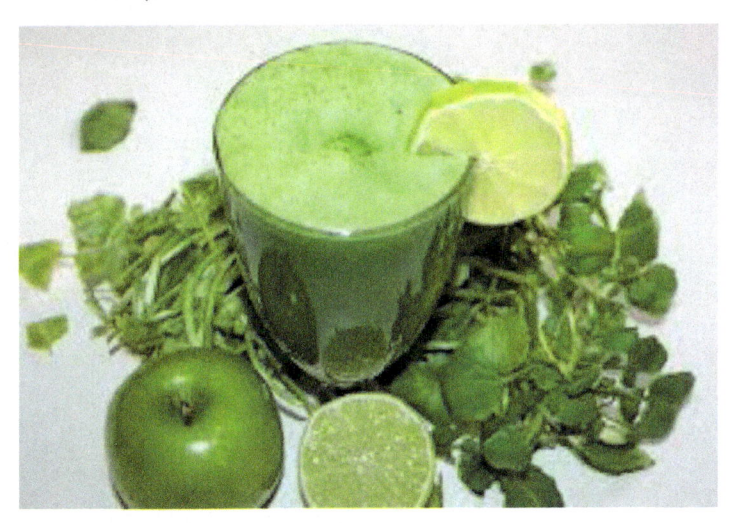

Preparation Time: 15 minutes

Servings: 4

Ingredients:

1/2 lemon, peeled

1/2 cucumber

Handful watercress

1/2 cup broccoli

1 green apple

1 kale stalk

1/2 fennel bulb

2 mint springs

1/2 cup blackberries

Directions:

Add all ingredients into the juicer and blend.

Lettuce Ginger Carrot Juice

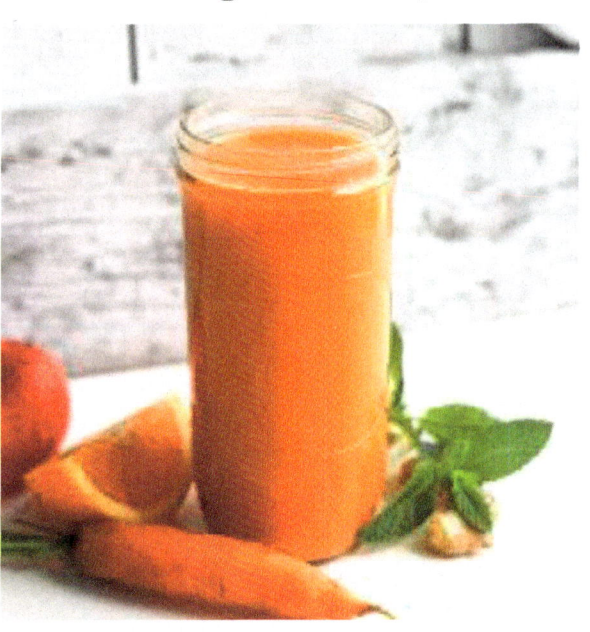

Preparation Time: 10 minutes

Servings: 4

Ingredients:

1 carrot

1 cup fresh parsley

1 bunch Swiss chard

1 lemon, peeled

1/2-inch fresh ginger

4 romaine lettuce leaves

1 green apple

Directions:

Add all ingredients into the juicer and blend.

Serve immediately and enjoy.

Spinach Orange Celery Juice

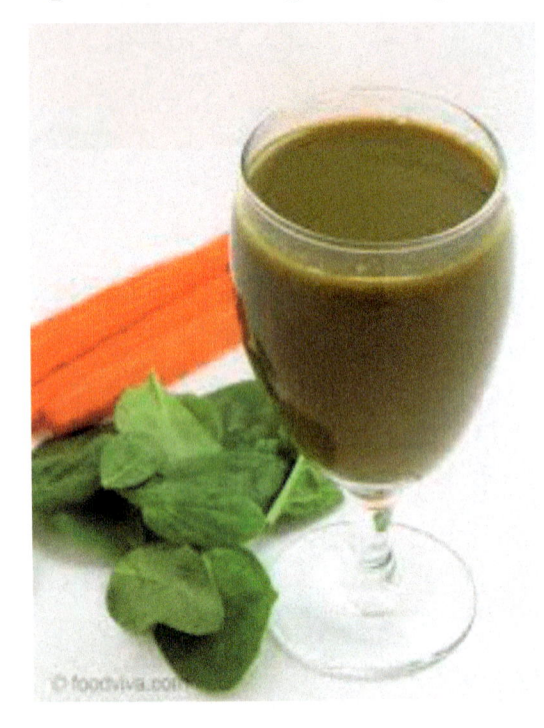

Preparation Time: 10 minutes

Servings: 4

Ingredients:

1 1/2 cups fresh spinach

1/2-inch fresh ginger

1 celery stalk

2 oranges, peeled

1 lime, peeled

2 lemons, peeled

1 green apple

Directions:

Add all ingredients into the juicer and blend.

Serve immediately and enjoy.

Fennel Dill Apple Juice

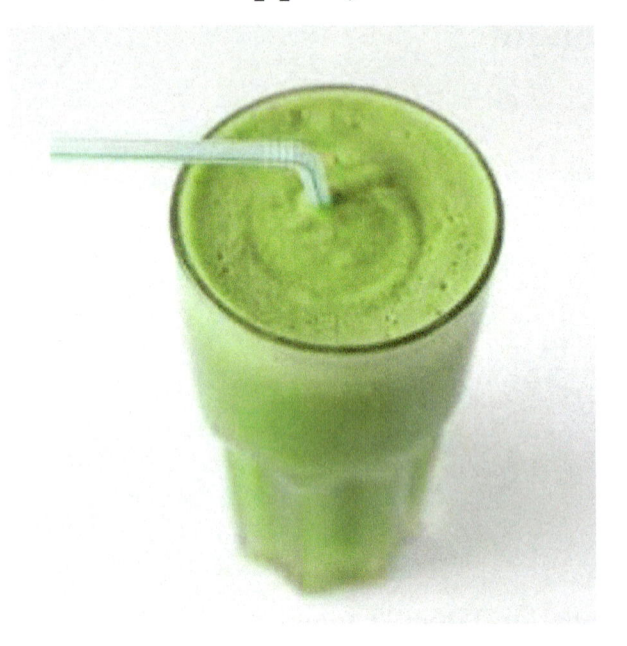

Preparation Time: 10 minutes

Servings: 4

Ingredients:

1/2 lemon, peeled

1 cucumber

2 green apples

4 tbsp fresh dill

1 cup baby spinach

2 fennel bulbs

Directions:

Add all ingredients into the juicer and blend.

Serve and enjoy.

Apple Strawberry Spinach Juice

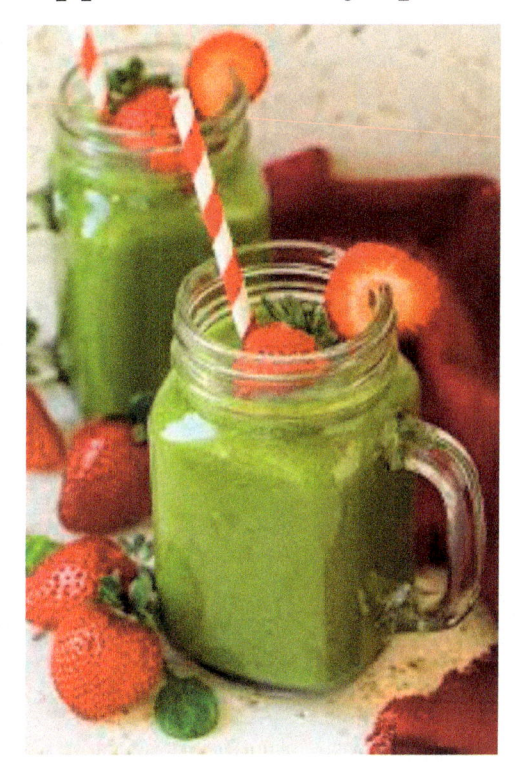

Preparation Time: 10 minutes

Servings: 4

Ingredients:

1 apple

Handful fresh parsley

Handful fresh spinach

10 strawberries

Directions:

Add all ingredients into the juicer and blend.

Serve and enjoy.

The Weight Loss Bunny Brew Juice

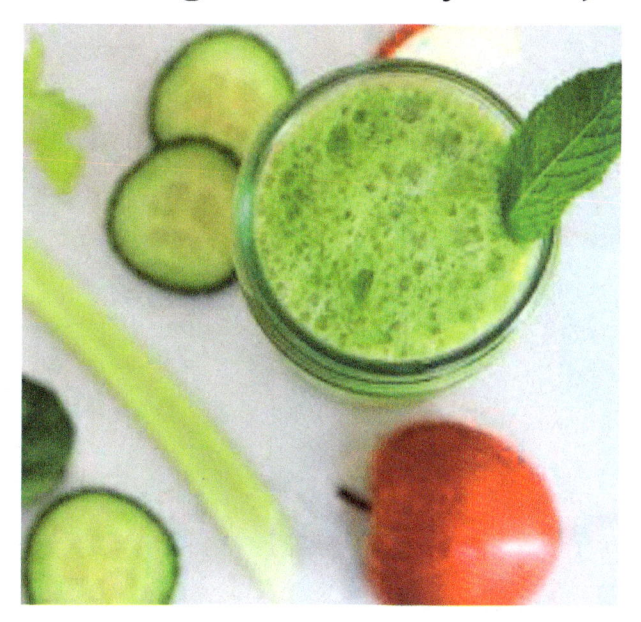

Preparation Time: 10 minutes

Servings: 4

Ingredients

7 medium carrots

½ a lemon

7 leaves of peppermint

½ of a pineapple fruit

Directions:

Add the ingredients to your juice.

Juice them thoroughly until you have a smooth juice.

Pour the drink into a glass and give it a nice shake.

Chill and serve!

The Cool Pink Pom Juice

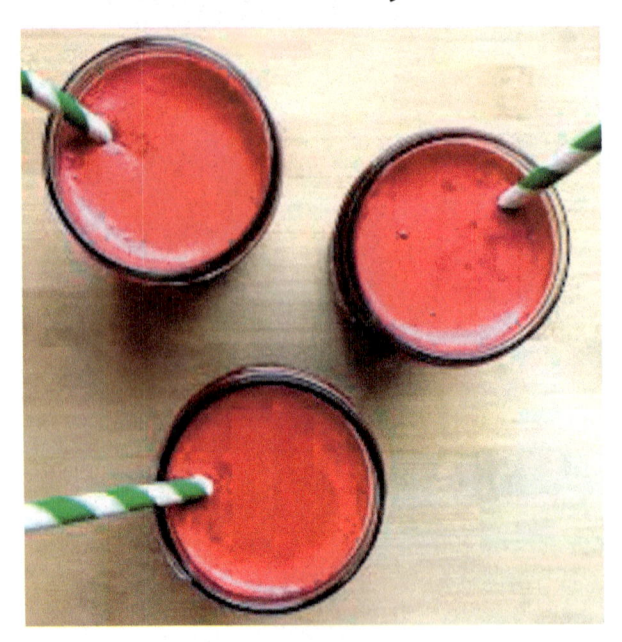

Preparation Time: 10 minutes

Servings: 4

Ingredients:

1 large apple of 3-inch diameter

½ of a thumb of ginger root 1-inch diameter

½ of a lemon fruit of 2-inch diameter

1 large orange fruit of 3-inch diameter

1 pomegranate of 4-inch diameter

Directions:

Add the ingredients to your juice.

Juice them thoroughly until you have a smooth juice.

Pour the drink into a glass and give it a nice shake.

Chill and serve!

The Mean Belly Buster Juice

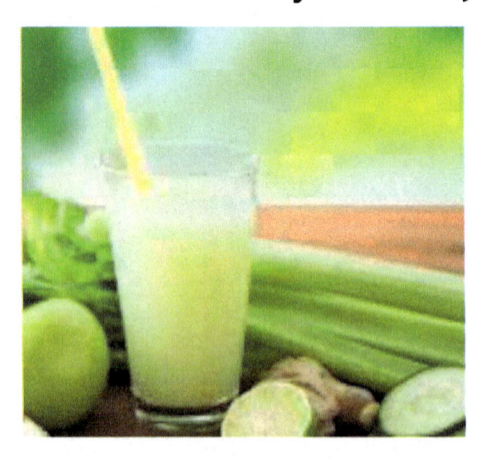

Preparation Time: 10 minutes

Servings: 4

Ingredients:

3 medium-sized Fuji apples

1 large cucumber

1 large lemon (with skin)

3 small mandarins (with skin)

1 romaine lettuce head

Directions:

Add the ingredients to your juicer/centrifuge

Juice them thoroughly until you have a smooth juice

Pour the drink into a glass and give it a nice shake

Chill and serve!

The Cellulite Fat Killer Juice

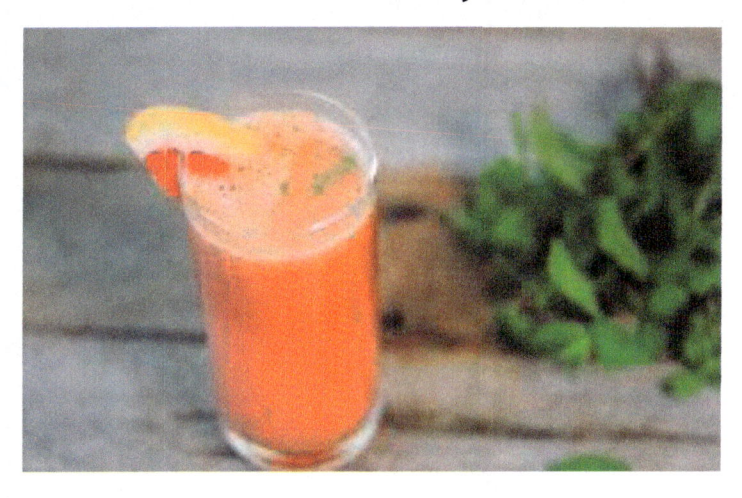

Preparation Time: 10 minutes

Servings: 4

Ingredients:

5 grapefruits

1 lemon fruit

2 limes

¼ of a medium-sized pineapple cut up into chunks

A handful of ginger

Directions:

Add the ingredients to your juicer.

Juice them thoroughly until you have a smooth juice.

Pour the drink into a glass and give it a nice shake.

Chill and serve!

Chapter 8: Juices for Energy Boosting

Brussels Green Juice

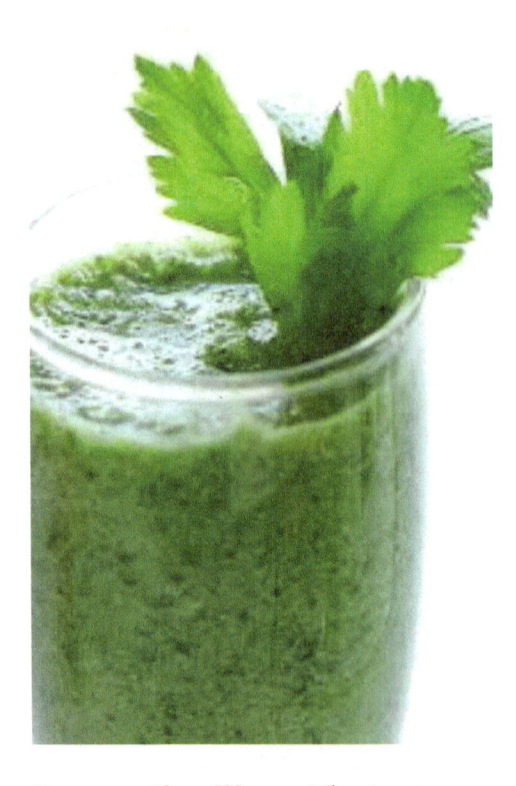

Preparation Time: 15 minutes

Servings: 5

Ingredients:

10 Brussels sprouts (3 cups chopped)

4 leaves Swiss chard

1 apple

Directions:

Juice all ingredients in the juicer, add ice if desired and it's ready to serve.

Green Pumpkin Smoothie

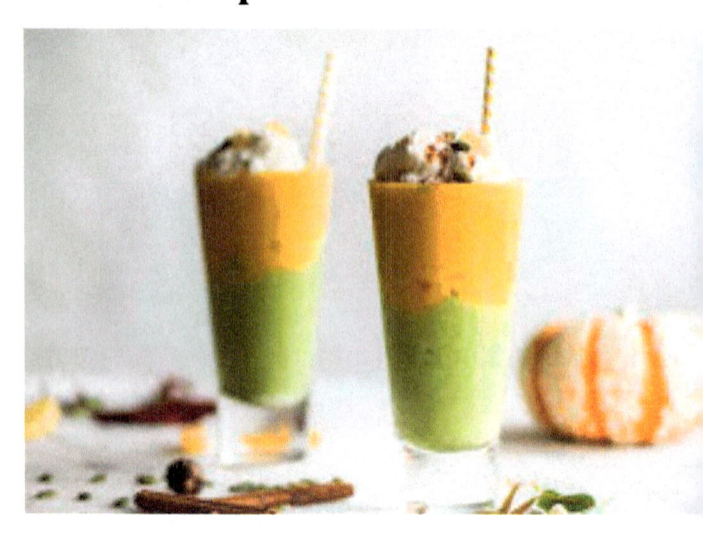

Preparation Time: 15 minutes

Servings: 5

Ingredients:

1/3 cup pumpkin puree

½ cup coconut milk

1/3 cup plain yogurt

½ teaspoon cinnamon

2 ripe bananas, sliced

1 cup fresh spinach leaves

Directions:

First, puree separately the pumpkin. When done, blend together with other fruits and vegetable ingredients.

Seven Green Giant Layers Juice

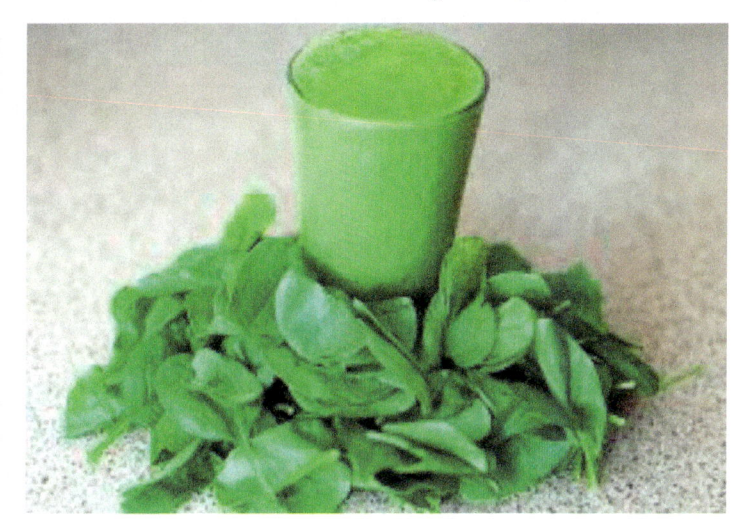

Preparation Time: 15 minutes

Servings: 5

Ingredients:

½ head fennel of leaves and bulb

¼ head green cabbage

3 stalks of celery

1 cucumber

1 green bell pepper

2 knuckles of ginger

1 sweet potato

Directions:

Juice all ingredients in the juicer, add ice if desired and it's ready to serve.

Breezy Green Juice

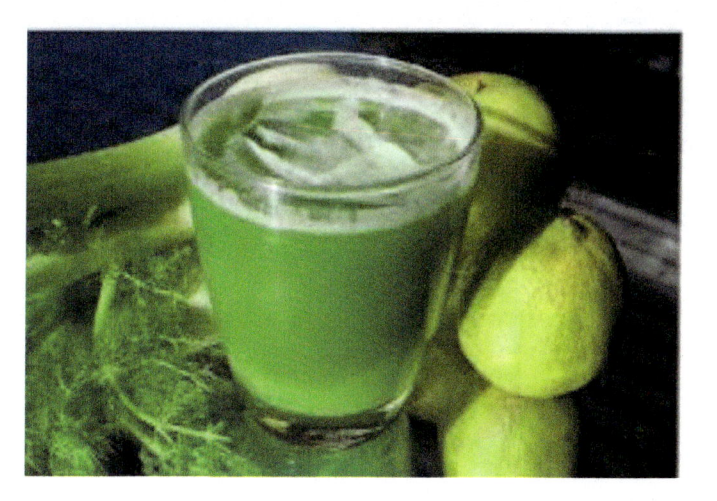

Preparation Time: 15 minutes

Servings: 5

Ingredients:

½ medium green cabbages

7 beet greens of stalks and leaves

1 stalk with leaves funnel

1/2 cucumbers

Directions:

Juice all ingredients in the juicer, add ice if desired and it's ready to serve.

Whole Green Goodness Juice

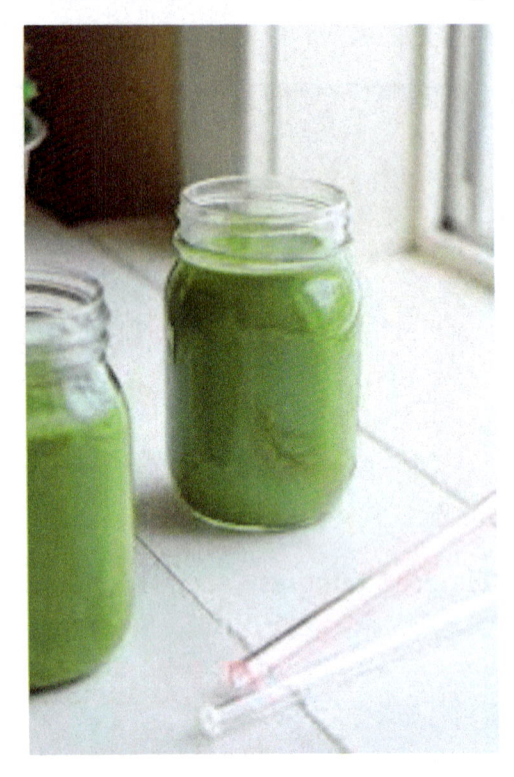

Preparation Time: 15 minutes

Servings: 5

Ingredients:

1/3 large bunch of spinach

5 stalks of celery

5 red leaves chard

4 leaves of kale

1 apple

1 head broccoli

Directions:

Juice all ingredients in the juicer, add ice if desired and it's ready to serve.

Ginger Pear Juice

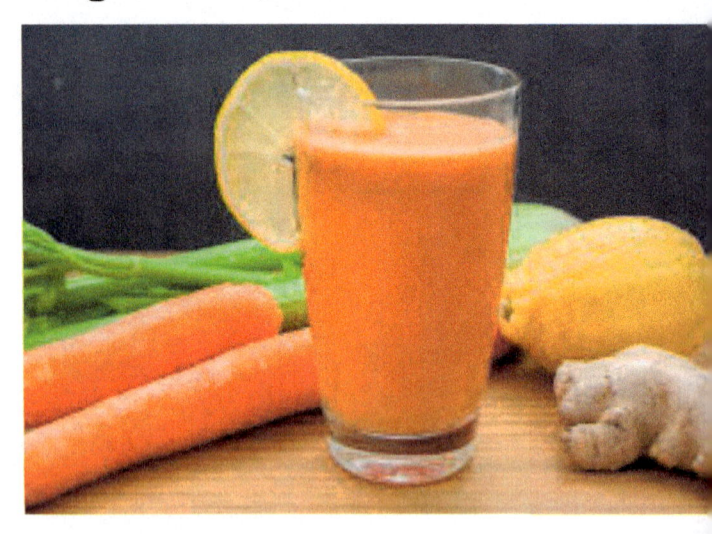

Preparation Time: 15 minutes

Servings: 2

Ingredients:

2 sprigs of fresh rosemary

6 leaves romaine lettuce

1 pear

1" fresh ginger root

2 celery roots (celeriac)

Directions

Peel ginger and celery roots then add to a juicer along with pear, rosemary, and romaine lettuce then juice. Serve immediately.

Apple Basil Kiwi Juice

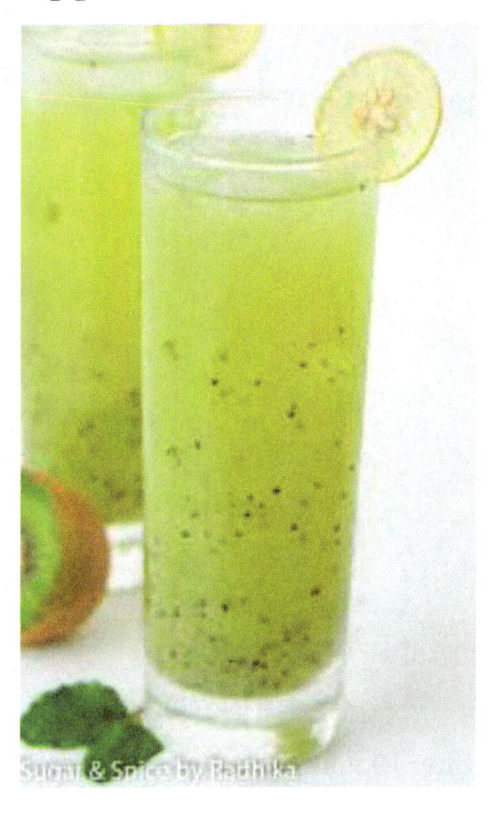

Preparation Time: 15 minutes

Servings: 2

Ingredients:

1 small container of strawberries

1 leaf and stalk of fennel

3 carrots

3 kiwis

Directions

Add the ingredients to a juicer and process into juice.

To help simplify the process, consider juicing the kiwi first, and then add in carrots, strawberries, and fennel.

You can skip the kiwi fruit or double the ingredients to make more juice.

Cranberry Pomegranate Juice

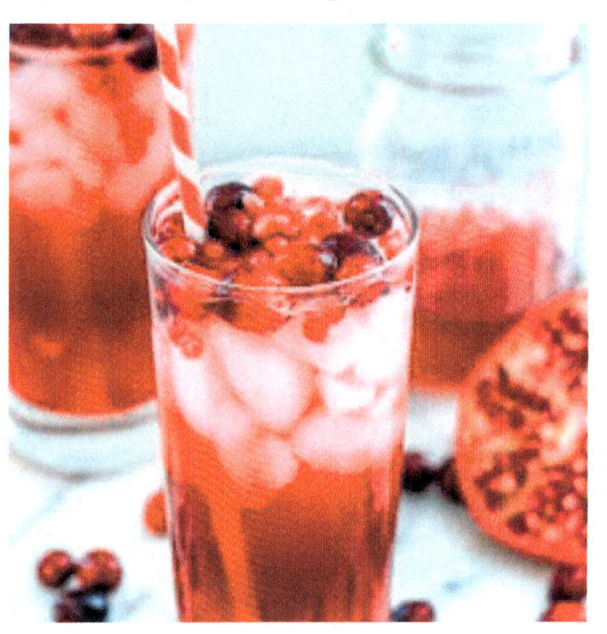

Preparation Time: 15 minutes

Servings: 2

Ingredients:

6 leaves fresh mint

1" fresh ginger root, peeled

1 pear, cored

1 cup cranberries

1 cup pomegranate seeds

6 large leaves kale

Directions

Push fresh mint, ginger, cranberries, kale, and pomegranate seeds through your juicer.

Discard the pulp then serve.

Energy Booster Green Juice

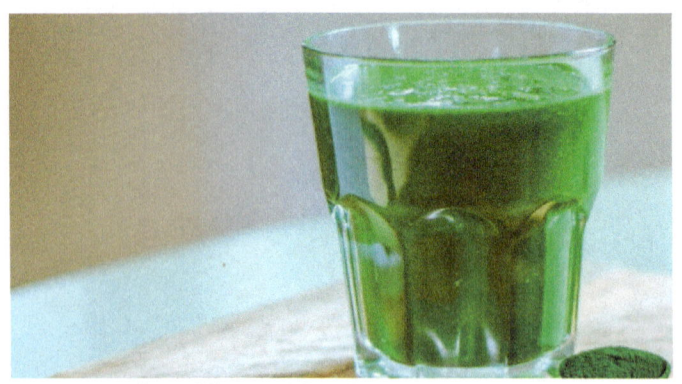

Preparation Time: 10 minutes

Servings: 4

Ingredients:

1/2 tsp spirulina powder

1 1/4 cups cold water

1/8 tsp salt

1 tsp stevia

1 lime juice

Handful mint

Handful spinach

1/2-inch fresh ginger

1/2 cucumber

1 kale leaf

1/2 green apple

1 celery stalk

Directions:

Juice all ingredients in the juicer, add ice if desired and it's ready to serve.

Green Peach Drink Juice

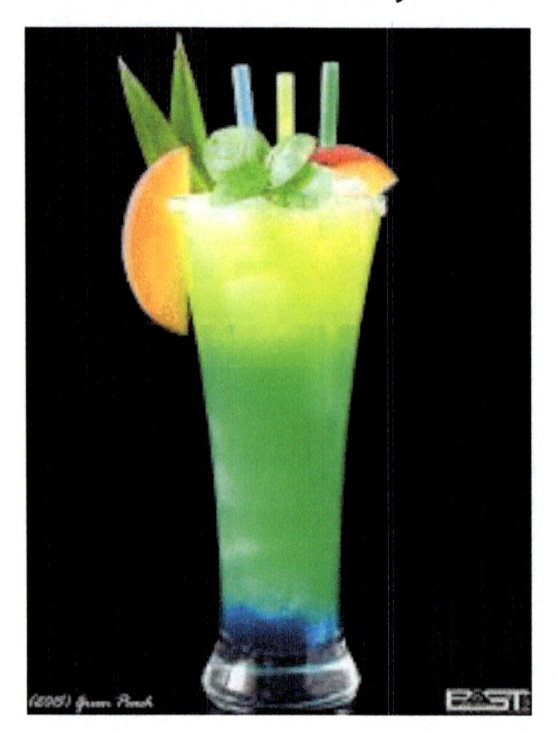

Preparation Time: 10 minutes

Servings: 2

Ingredients:

1 peach, pitted

3 kale leaves

2 medium carrots

1 slice ginger, peeled

Directions:

Add the peach, kale leaves, carrots, and ginger into a juicer. Stir the juice before serving.

Coconut and Litchi Juice

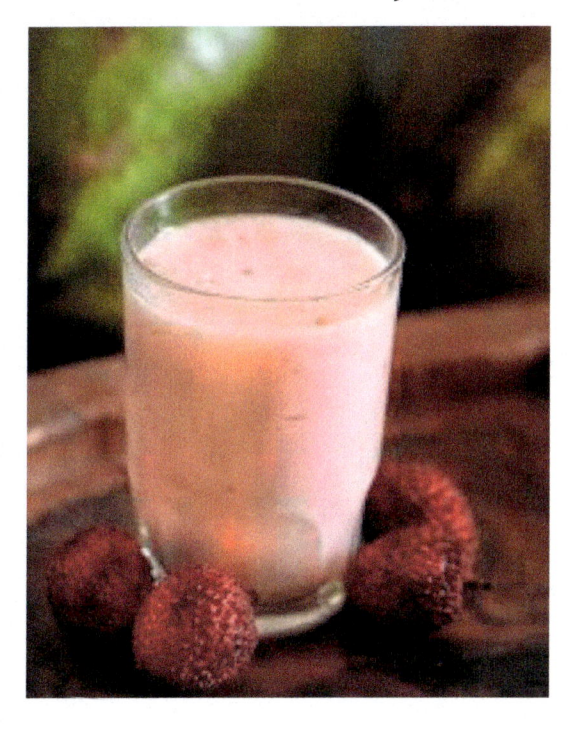

Preparation Time: 10 minutes

Servings: 2

Ingredients:

1 cup coconut water

25 litchis (peeled and seeds removed)

1 cup peaches (sliced)

Directions:

Push all the ingredients through the juicer and juice.

Goji Berry Juice

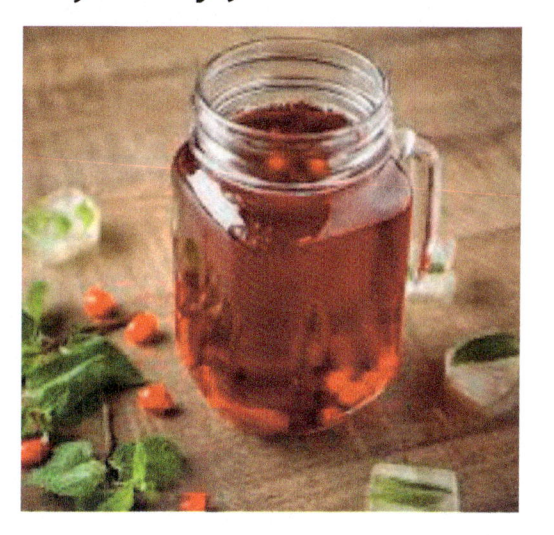

Preparation Time: 10 minutes

Servings: 2

Ingredients:

46 oz pineapple Juice.

2.8 oz goji berries.

Directions:

Place the goji berries in the pineapple juice for 24 hours to rehydrate.

Transfer into a blender and blend.

Strain the juice and refrigerate to chill.

Wheatgrass Carrot Juice

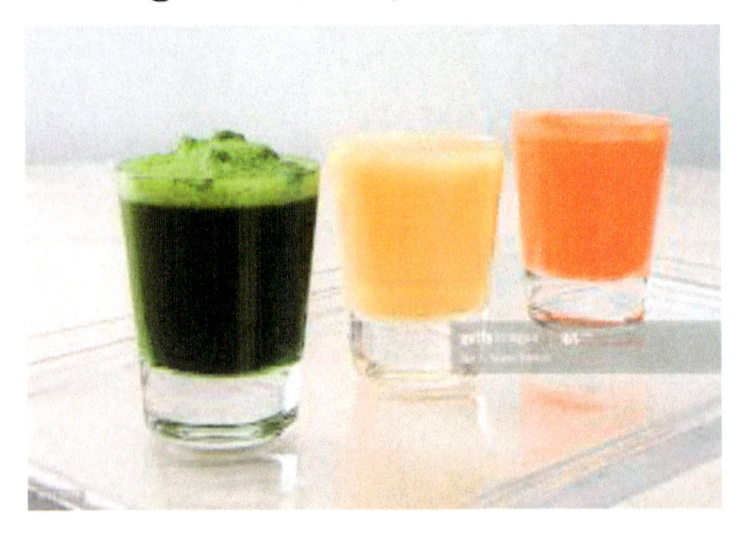

Preparation Time: 10 minutes

Servings: 2

Ingredients:

2 green apples

3 sprigs fresh mint

1/4 lime, peeled

2 carrots

2 handfuls wheatgrass

Directions:

Juice the apples, mint, lime, carrot, and wheatgrass.

Discard the pulp and serve.

Avocado Sprout Smoothie

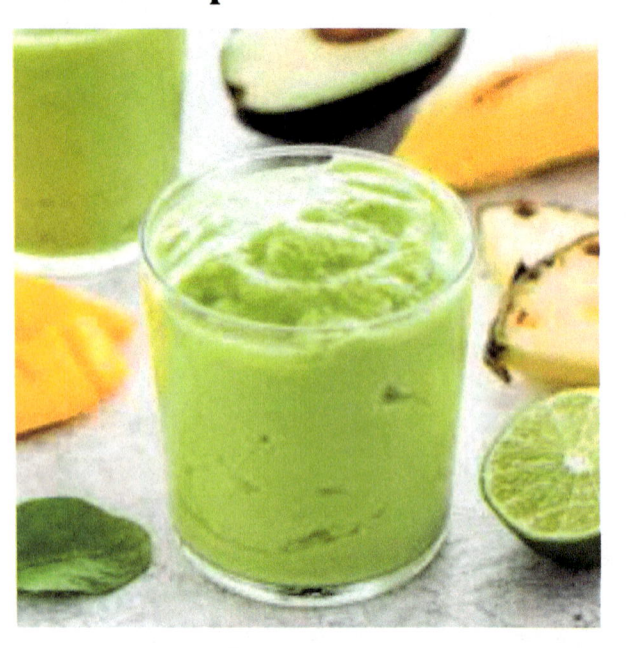

Preparation Time: 15 minutes

Servings: 5

Ingredients

1 tablespoon fresh mint leaves

Dash of salt

Dash of cayenne pepper

1 cup of soy milk

1 tablespoon lime juice

1 medium-sized avocado, peeled and sliced

1 tablespoon honey

½ cup sprouts

Directions:

Mix all ingredients into the blender and blend until smooth and creamy.

Energizer Juice

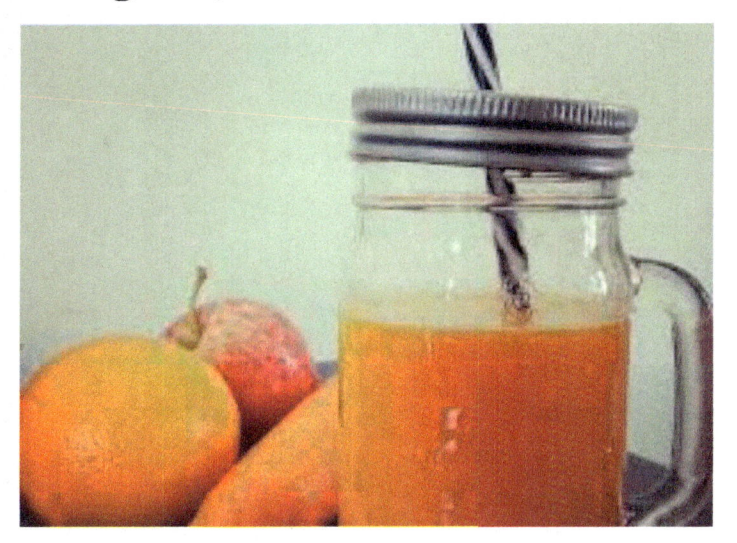

Preparation Time: 10 minutes

Servings: 4

Ingredients:

1 oz chopped kale

1 apple

1-kiwi

½ cucumber

½ cup spinach

5 parsley sprigs

½ lemon

½ oz ginger

Directions:

Push all the ingredients through the juicer and juice.

Strawberry and Apple Juice

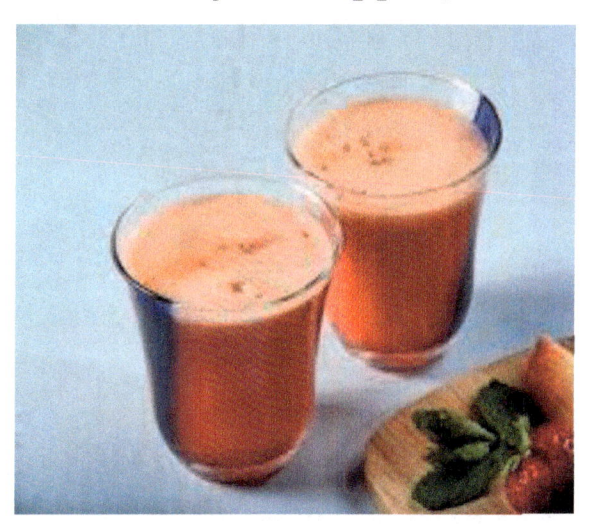

Preparation Time: 15 minutes

Servings: 5

Ingredients:

1 red apple (chopped)

1 punnet strawberries

Directions:

Push all the ingredients through the juicer and juice.

Serve chilled.

Beet Martini Juice

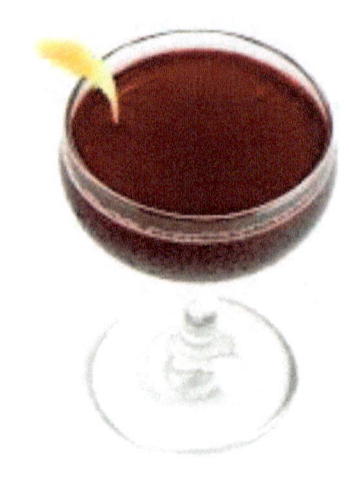

Preparation Time: 10 minutes

Servings: 2

Ingredients:

1 beet, peeled

1-ounce vodka

1 small red apple

1 orange, peeled

1 thin orange wedge

4 mint leaves

Ice cubes

Direction:

Juice the beet, apple, and orange. Place the juice and vodka into a shaker with ice cubes and shake well. Rub the mint leaves on the rim of a martini glass. Pour the juice and vodka mixture into the martini glass. Garnish the drink with an orange wedge and a few mint leaves.

Cabbage Patch Juice

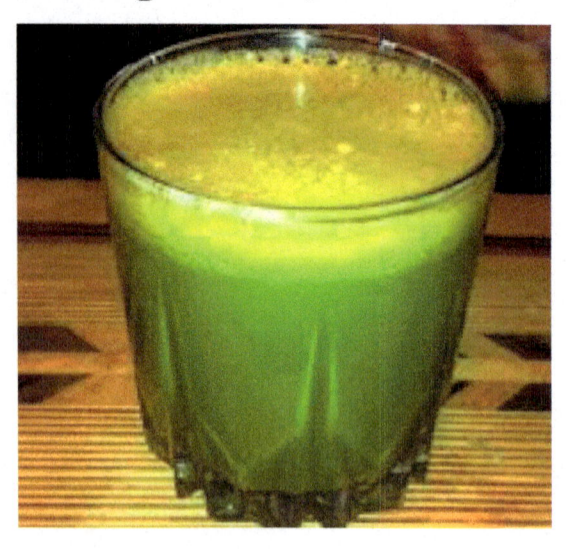

Preparation Time: 10 minutes

Servings: 2

Ingredients:

8 cabbage leaves

8 kale leaves

3 medium carrots

1 pear

1-inch ginger

Directions:

Process the cabbage, kale, carrots, pear, and ginger in a juicer and mix well.

Cognition Booster Juice

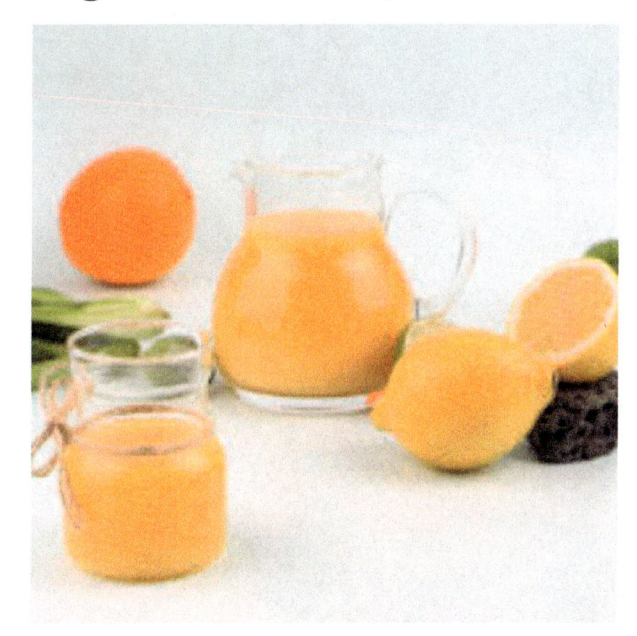

Preparation Time: 15 minutes

Servings: 2

Ingredients:

3 medium carrots

1 sweet potato

1 beetroot

Directions

Juice the carrots, sweet potato, and beetroot

Pour into a glass and enjoy.

Cilantro Apple Green Juice

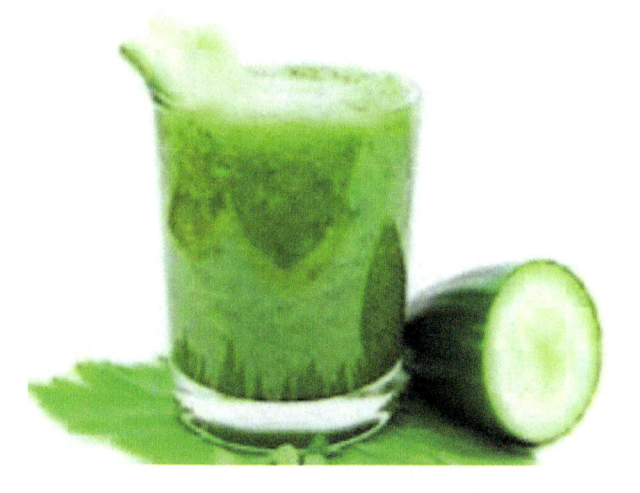

Preparation Time: 15 minutes

Servings: 2

Ingredients:

½ lemon, peeled

¼ cup fresh cilantro

1 medium cucumber

2 large kale leaves

2 stalks celery

2 green apples

Directions

Gather all the ingredients then press them through a juicer.

Stir the juice then serve and enjoy.

Pineapple Cucumber Kale Juice

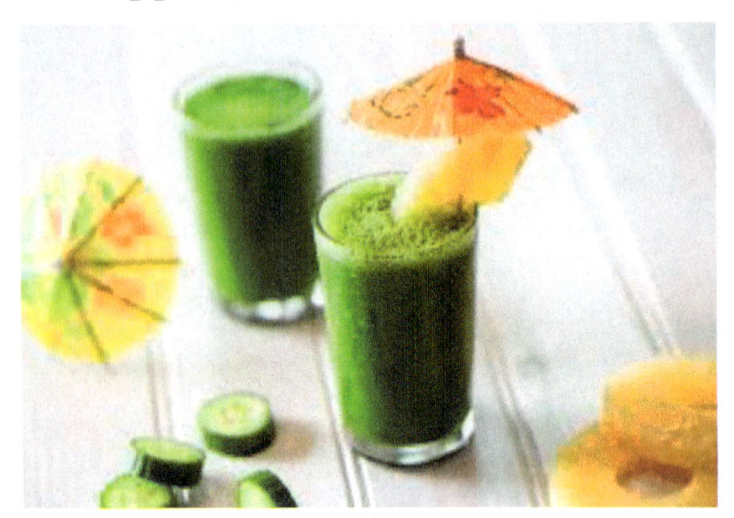

Preparation Time: 10 minutes

Servings: 2

Ingredients:

2 cups tightly packed kale

2 cucumbers

2 cups fresh pineapple

Directions:

Add the following ingredients to your juicer.

Process to obtain the juice. Serve and enjoy.

Banana Berry Smoothie

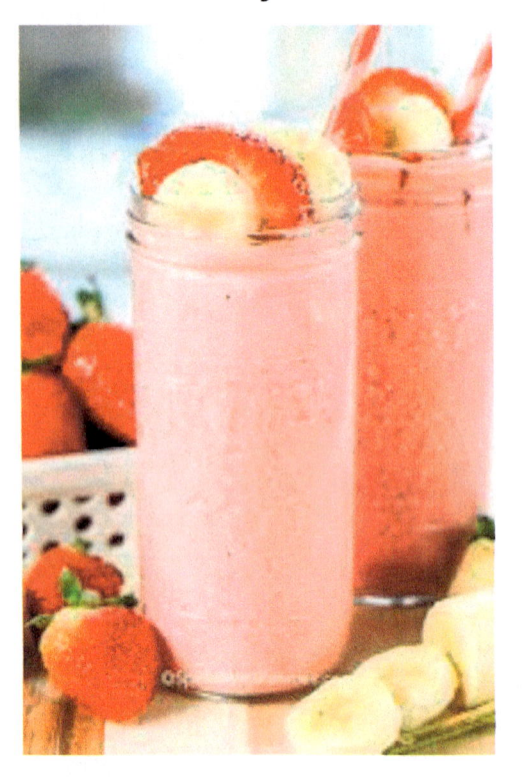

Preparation Time: 15 minutes

Servings: 5

Ingredients:

1 cup spinach

1 cup pure water

1 cup sliced bananas

1 cup fresh blueberries

Directions:

Mix all ingredients into the blender and blend until smooth and creamy.

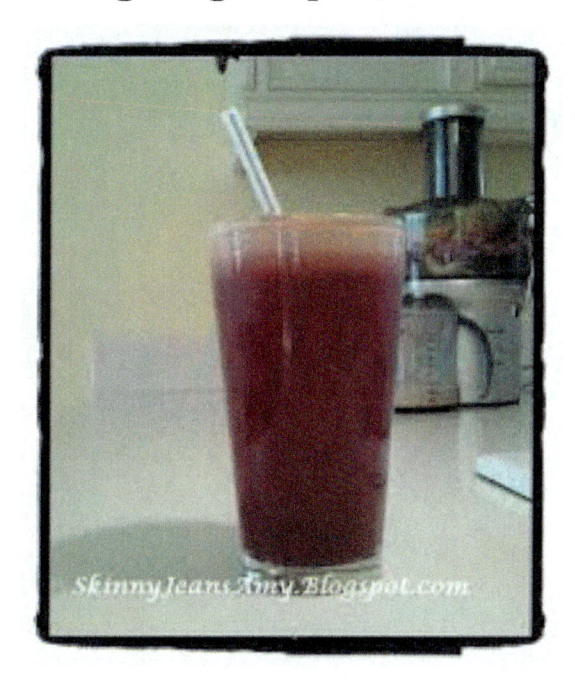

Energizing Purple Juice

Preparation Time: 15 minutes

Servings: 5

Ingredients:

2 carrots (peeled)

½ red cabbage (chopped)

1 apple

½ lemon

¼ cantaloupe Melon (skin removed, chopped)

Directions:

Add all the ingredients to the juicer and juice.

Masterpiece of Green Goodness Juice

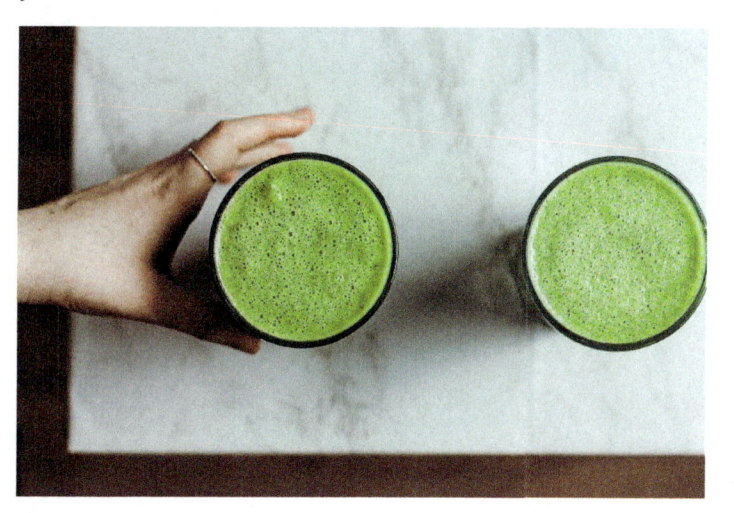

Preparation Time: 15 minutes

Servings: 5

Ingredients:

3 leaves kale

1/3 small bunch cilantro

6 carrots

3 radishes leaves and radish

1 cucumber

1 green cabbage

1 green pepper

Directions:

Juice all ingredients in the juicer, add ice if desired and it's ready to serve.

Amazing Sunflower Greens Smoothie

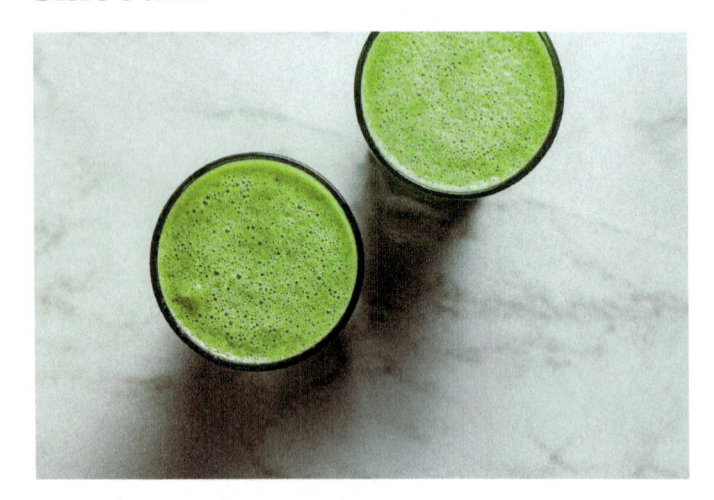

Preparation Time: 15 minutes

Servings: 5

Ingredients:

1 cup alfalfa

1 carrot, peeled and sliced

1 red apple, unpeeled and sliced

1 tablespoon agave

1 cup sunflower greens

1 cup kale

Directions:

Mix all ingredients into the blender and blend until smooth and creamy.

Green Tango Juice

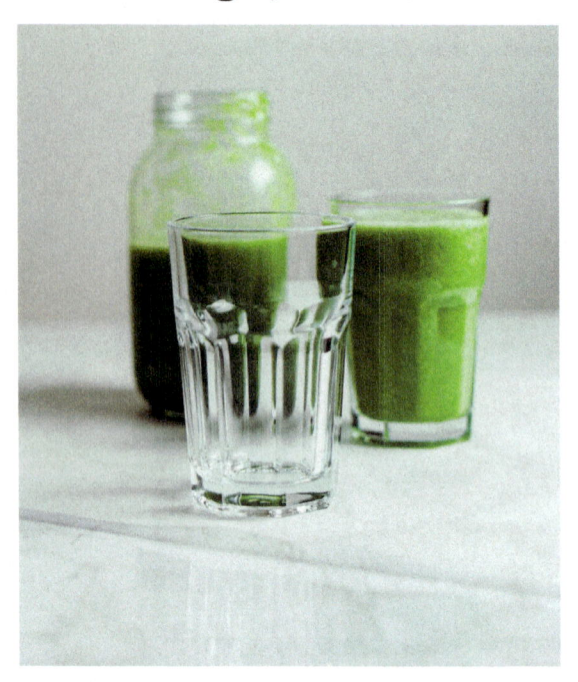

Preparation Time: 15 minutes

Servings: 5

Ingredients:

4 leaves kale

4 stalks of celery

1/3 small bunch of spinach

1 large apple

1 knuckle ginger

Directions:

Juice all ingredients in the juicer, add ice if desired and it's ready to serve.

Energetic Litchi Blueberry Juice

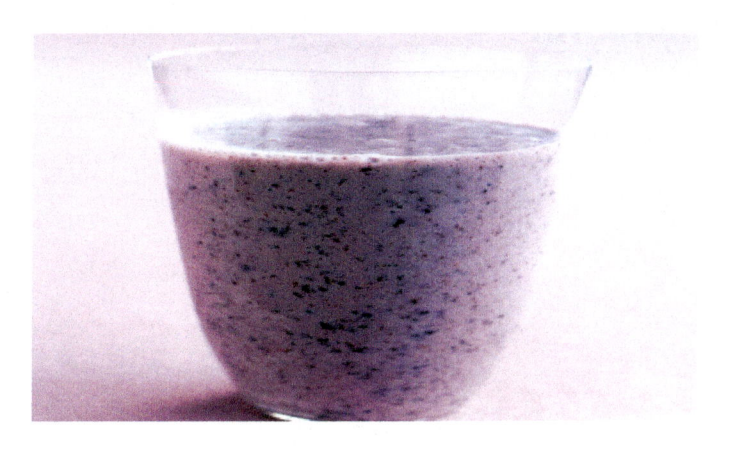

Preparation Time: 10 minutes

Servings: 4

Ingredients:

1 cup litchi

1/2 cup fresh blueberries

1/8 tsp salt

1 handful mint leaves

1 tbsp lime juice

Directions:

Add all ingredients into the juicer and blend.

Serve and enjoy.

Morning Buzz Juice

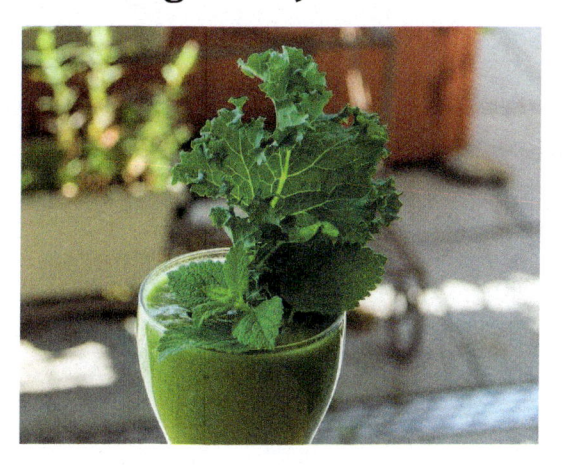

Preparation Time: 15 minutes

Servings: 5

Ingredients:

1 pear

10 leaves kale

1 knuckle ginger

Directions:

Juice all ingredients in the juicer, add ice if desired and it's ready to serve.

Hot Green Lover Juice

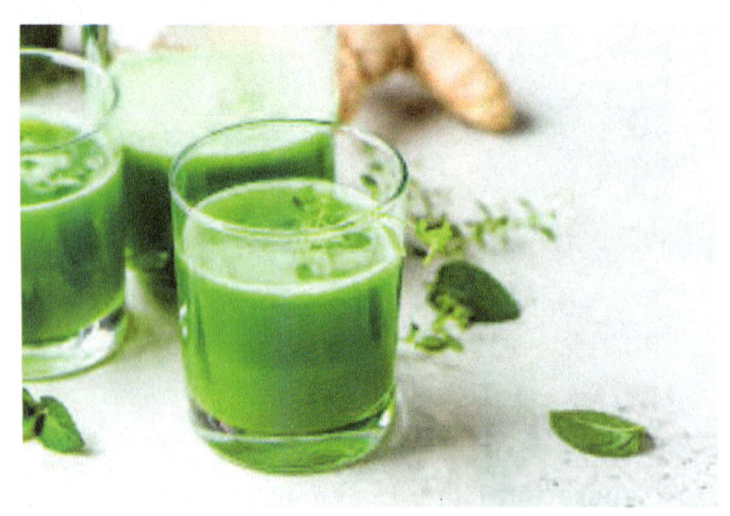

Preparation Time: 15 minutes

Servings: 5

Ingredients:

4 leaves of collard greens

4 leaves of Swiss chard

1 green cabbage

1 knuckle ginger

Directions:

Juice all ingredients in the juicer, add ice if desired and it's ready to serve.

Pineapple, Banana, and Kale Smoothie

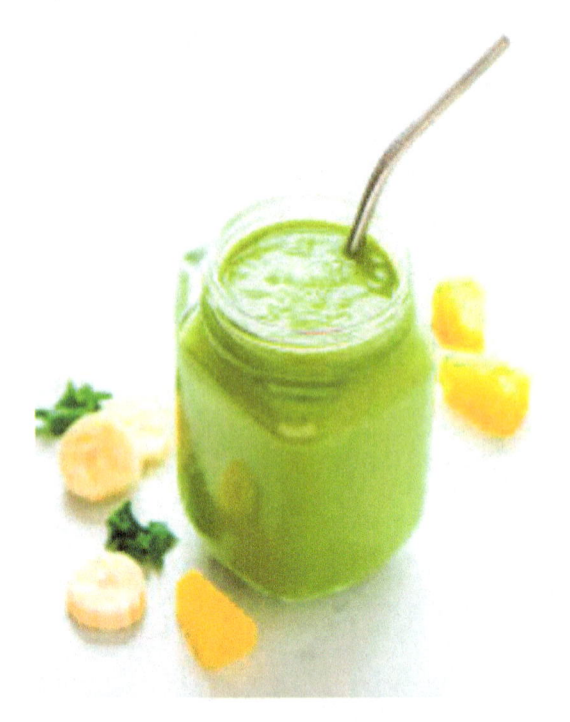

Preparation Time: 15 minutes

Servings: 5

Ingredients:

1 ½ cup of sliced pineapple of medium size

½ cup coconut milk

2 cups hashed kale

1 full grown banana sliced into medium size

Directions:

Add together 1 ½ cup of sliced pineapple, ½ cup coconut milk, 2 cups hashed kale, and 1 sliced banana.

Ginger Power Smoothie

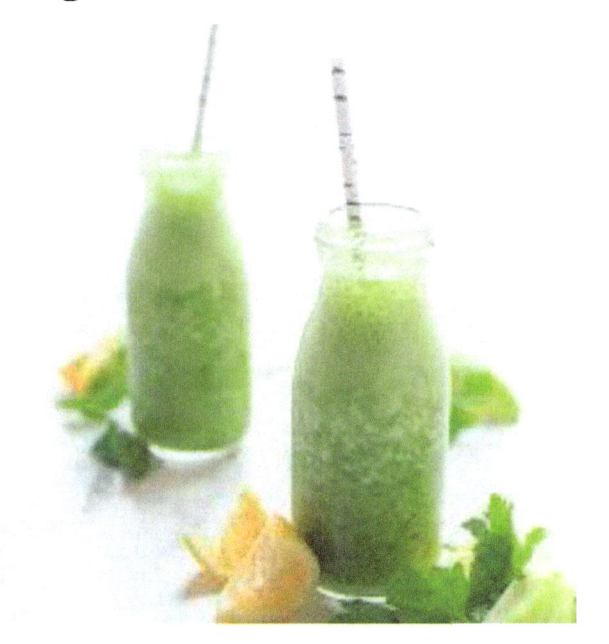

Preparation Time: 15 minutes

Servings: 5

Ingredients:

1 lemon, unpeeled and sliced

1 tablespoon ginger, unpeeled and sliced thinly

8 leaves of romaine lettuce, chopped

6 cups baby spinach, chopped

2 red apples, unpeeled and sliced

1/3 cup cucumber, unpeeled and sliced

2-3 garlic cloves, chopped thinly

Directions:

Jumble all ingredients together leaving the garlic last to blend. Start with mixing 1 garlic clove first and adjust the quantity as you feel appropriate to your taste.

Green Dream Juice

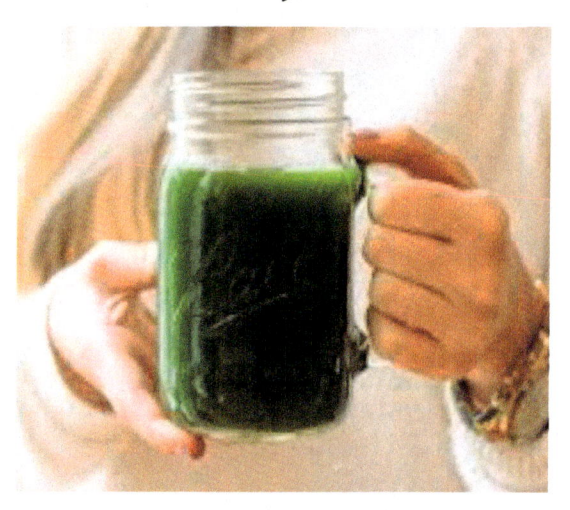

Preparation Time: 15 minutes

Servings: 5

Ingredients:

4 Leaves kale

3 Apples

1 Zucchini

1 head of broccoli

Directions:

Juice all ingredients in the juicer, add ice if desired and it's ready to serve.

Green Avocado Smoothie

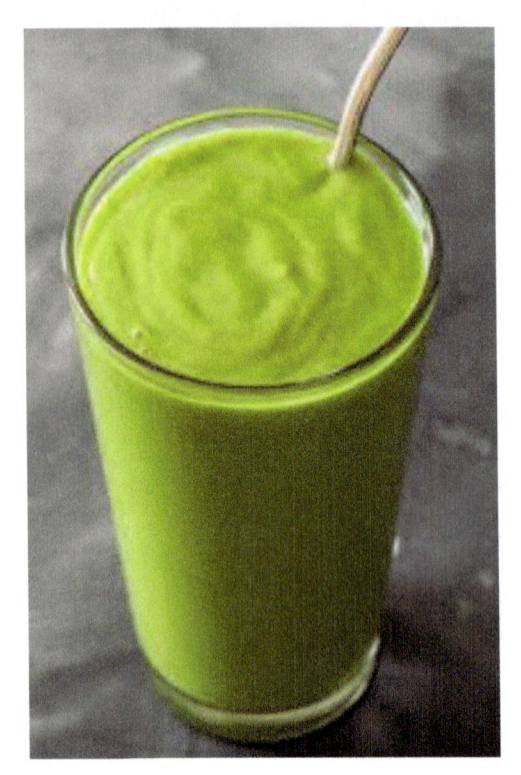

Preparation Time: 15 minutes

Servings: 5

Ingredients:

1 cup spinach

1 ¼ cup soy milk

½ medium avocado, peeled and chopped

½ cup fresh mango

1 ripe banana

½ teaspoon honey

Directions:

Mix all ingredients into the blender and blend until smooth and creamy.

Berry Cauliflower Smoothie

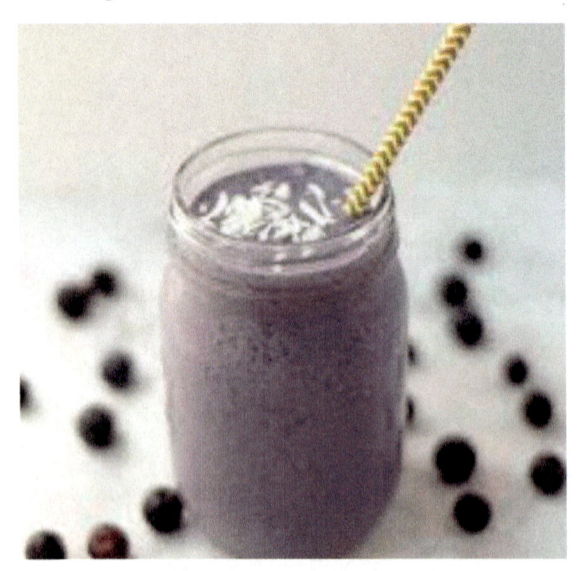

Preparation Time: 15 minutes

Servings: 5

Ingredients:

1 tablespoon chia seeds

5 ripe bananas, sliced

1 ½ cups cauliflower

1 cup pure water

12-ounce fresh strawberries

Directions:

Mix all ingredients into the blender and blend until smooth and creamy.

Pineapple Wheatgrass Smoothie

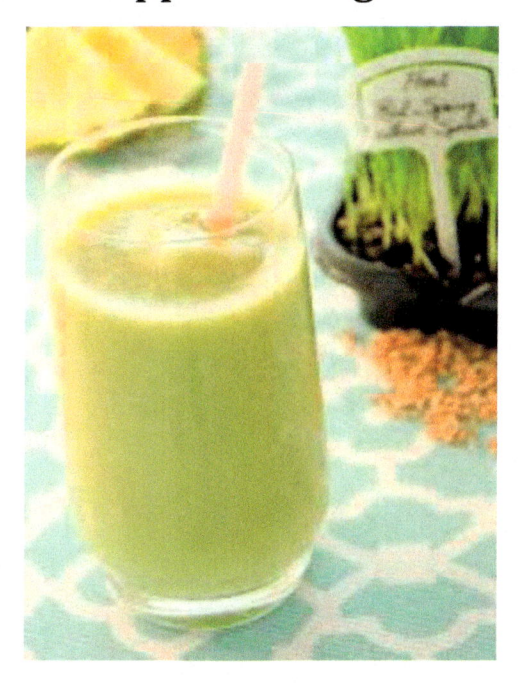

Preparation Time: 15 minutes

Servings: 5

Ingredients:

1 cup fresh pineapple, peeled and chopped

½ cold water

2 cups wheatgrass or wheatgrass juice

1 carrot, peeled and sliced

1 scoop wheatgrass powder

1 tablespoon lemon juice

1 tablespoon agave

Directions:

Mix all ingredients into the blender and blend until smooth and creamy.

Holy Kale Cleanse Juice

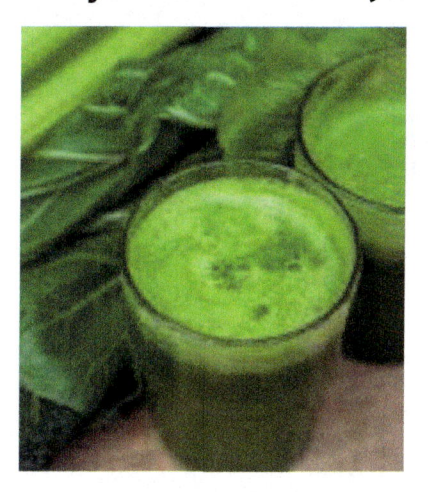

Preparation Time: 10 minutes

Servings: 2

Ingredients:

1 cup loosely packed fresh mint

2 oz. apple cider vinegar

1 1/2 apple

2" fresh ginger root

1/2 cucumber

1 bunch parsley

1 bunch kale

1/2 cup diced pineapple

1 lemon, peeled

Directions

Add all the ingredients to a juicer and press to extract the juice.

Stir the mixture then pour into a tall glass. Serve instantly and enjoy.

Very Berry Smoothie

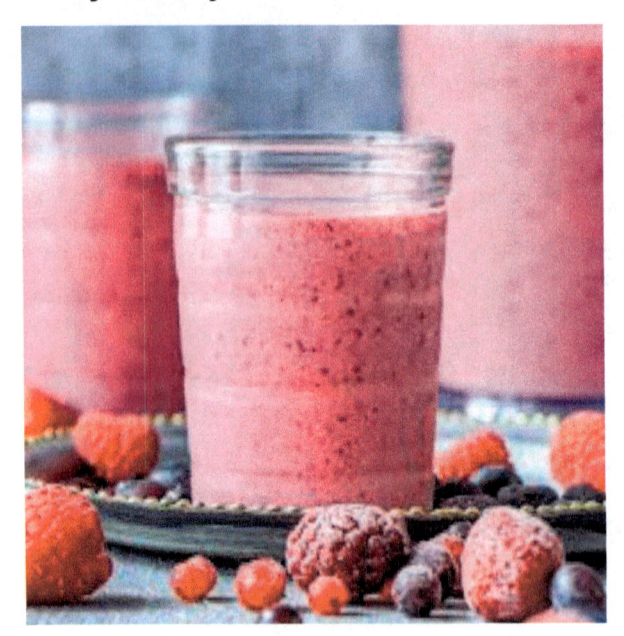

Preparation Time: 15 minutes

Servings: 5

Ingredients:

1 tablespoon honey

1 ½ cups of mixed berries (blueberries, mulberries, blackberries, strawberries)

¼ cup almond milk

½ cup ice cube

1 cup Greek yogurt

Directions:

Mix all ingredients in the blender until smooth.

Green Dawn Juice

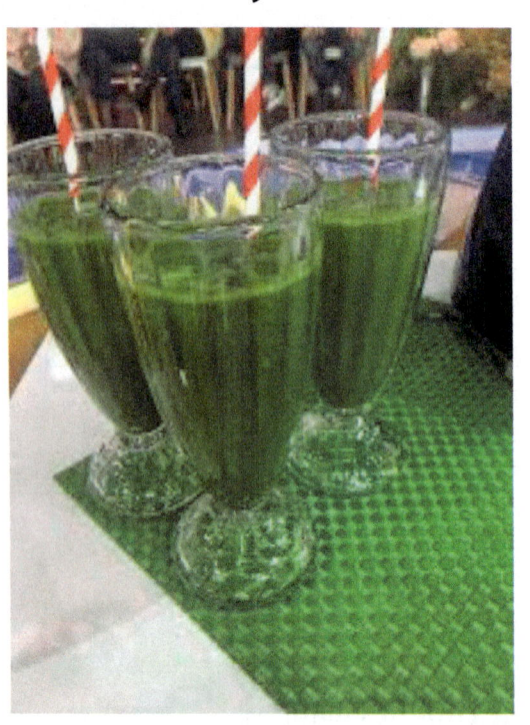

Preparation Time: 15 minutes

Servings: 5

Ingredients:

4 medium-sized carrots

4 romaine lettuce leaves

3 large rainbow chard leaves

1/2 cup bunch of spinach

1 small apple

1 knuckle of ginger (1 square inch)

Directions:

Juice all ingredients in the juicer, add ice if desired and it's ready to serve. You can add a little apple to make it sweet.

Grape Dates Green Smoothie

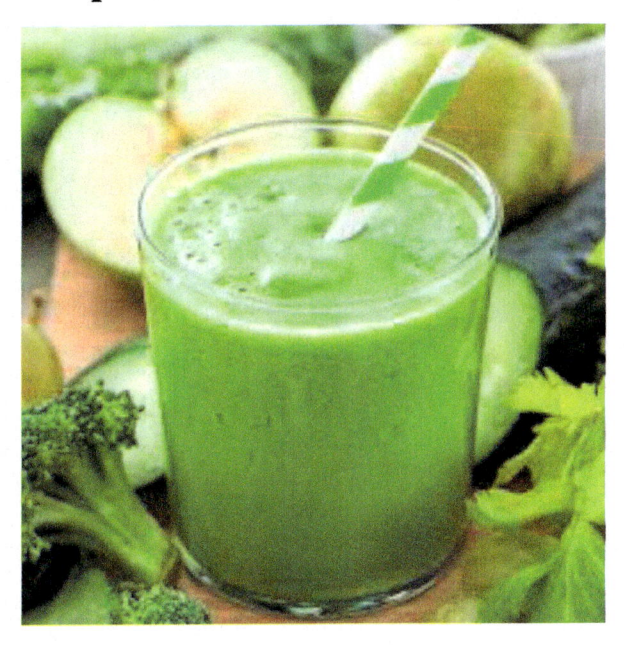

Preparation Time: 15 minutes

Servings: 5

Ingredients:

1 cup sliced grapes

1 medium-sized date

1/2 cup fresh spinach

1 cup coconut water

Directions:

Mix all ingredients into the blender and blend until smooth and creamy.

Power Jumble Smoothie

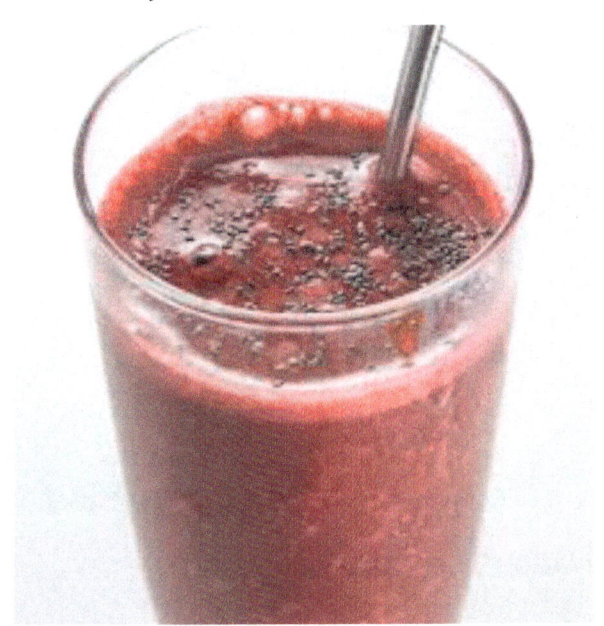

Preparation Time: 15 minutes

Servings: 5

Ingredients:

1 cup cabbage greens, chopped thinly

1 cup pineapple juice

1 cup sliced carrots

½ cup mint leaves

1 freshly squeezed lemon juice

1 cup cherry tomatoes

Directions:

Mix all ingredients into the blender and blend until smooth and creamy.

Three C's Juice

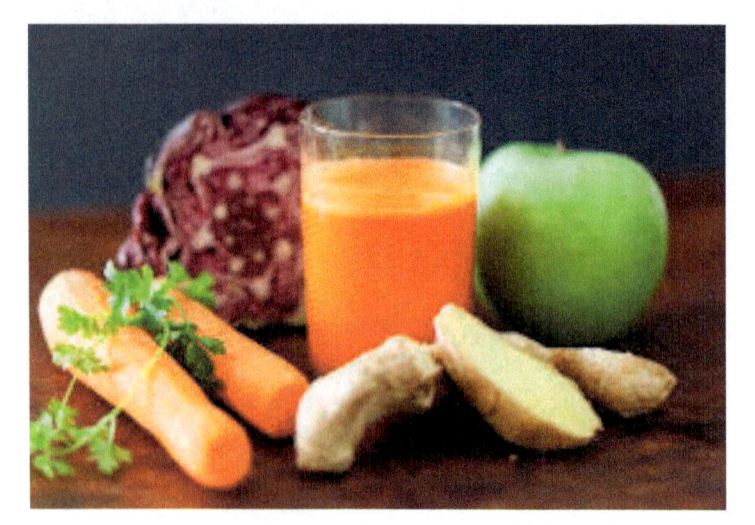

Preparation Time: 10 minutes

Servings: 2

Ingredients:

½ head green cabbage

7 medium carrots

7 celery stalks

2 green apples

1 lime

1-inch ginger

Ice cubes

Directions:

Place all the ingredients into a juicer and process until juices are extracted. Fill a glass halfway with ice cubes. Pour the juice over the ice and enjoy.

Spicy Orange Surprise Juice

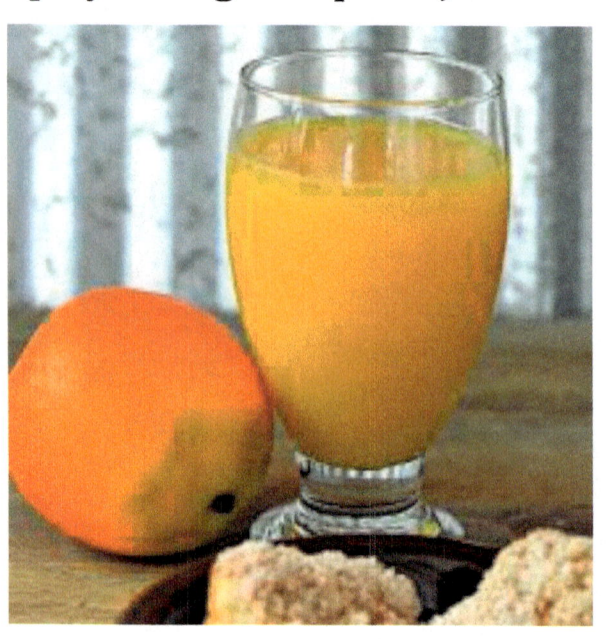

Preparation Time: 10 minutes

Servings: 2

Ingredients:

2 inches fresh turmeric

1 small zucchini

3 oranges

3 sweet potatoes

Directions:

Place all the ingredients into a juicer and process. Mix well before serving.

Blood Orange Juice

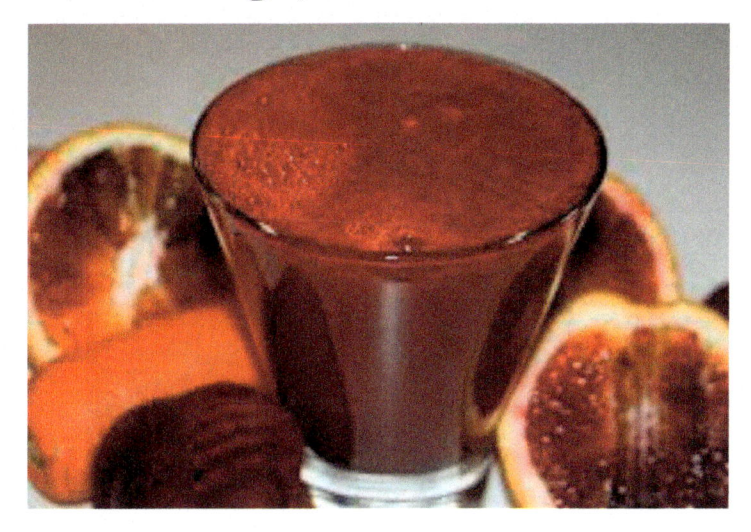

Preparation Time: 10 minutes

Servings: 2

Ingredients:

2 blood oranges, peeled

1 sweet potato, peeled

1 purple carrot

1 cup raspberries

2 celery sticks

Ice cubes

Directions:

Put the blood oranges, sweet potato, purple carrot, raspberries, and celery into a juicer. Place the juice and a few ice cubes into a shaker and shake well. Pour the juice into a glass and serve.

Purple Passion Juice

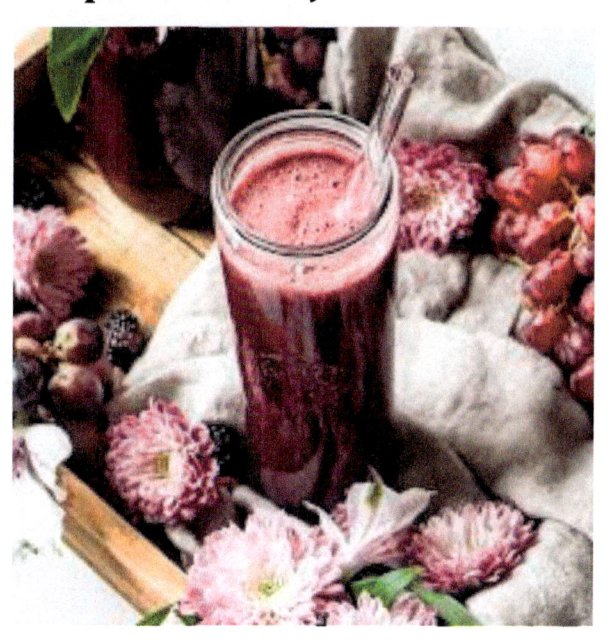

Preparation Time: 10 minutes

Servings: 2

Ingredients:

2 cups blackberries

2 cups red grapes

½ lemon fruit

Ice cubes

Directions:

Process the blackberries, red grapes, and lemon in a juicer. Pour the juice over a few ice cubes and enjoy!

The Green Clean Pineapple Juice

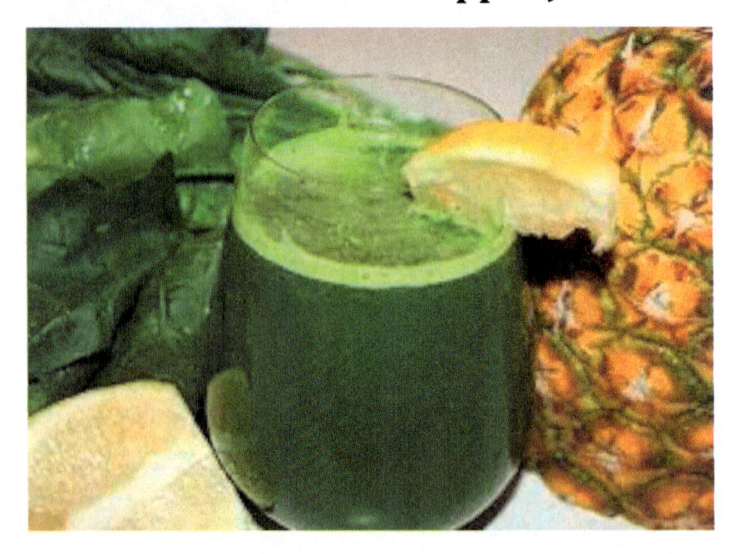

Preparation Time: 15 minutes

Servings: 2

Ingredients:

¾ cup fresh pineapple

3 cups baby spinach

3 tablespoons fresh ginger

1 cucumber

Directions:

Add all the ingredients to the juicer and juice.

Lime and Honeydew Melon Juice

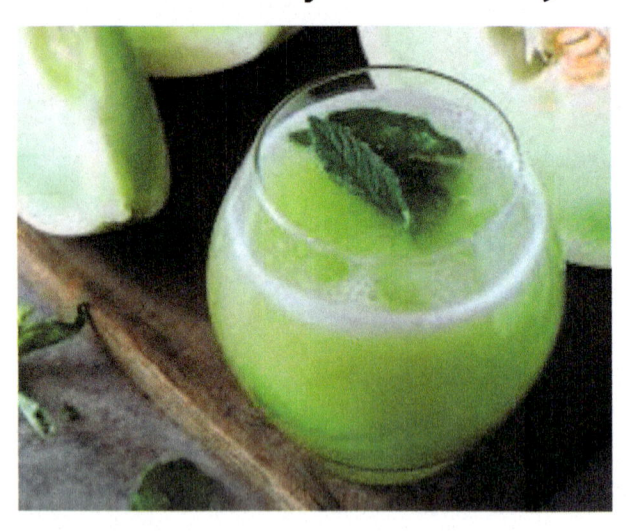

Preparation Time: 10 minutes

Servings: 2

Ingredients:

¼ honeydew melon (seeds and skin removed, chopped)

½ cucumber (chopped)

1 lime (skin and seeds removed)

Directions:

Add all the ingredients to the juicer and juice.

Pear Juice

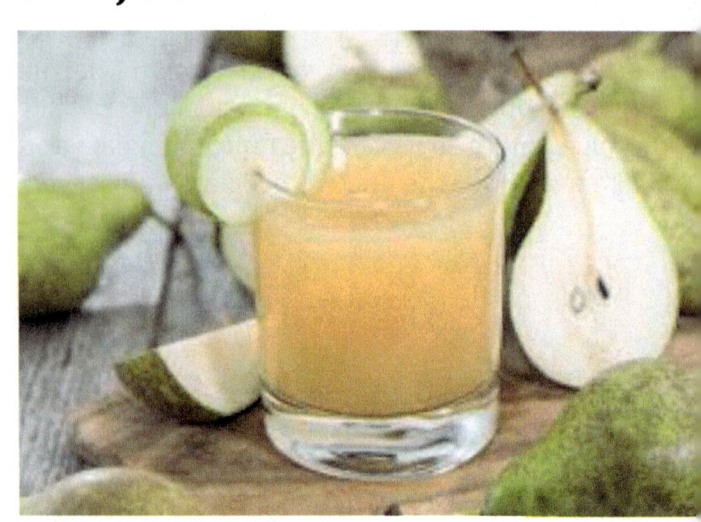

Preparation Time: 10 minutes

Servings: 2

Ingredients:

1 sweet Potato

2 pears

1 apple

1 1/3 cups blueberries

Just a dash of cinnamon

Directions:

Add all the ingredients to the juicer and juice.

Conclusion

I hope this book was able to help you discover the wonderful benefits of juicing and how it can effectively help you achieve long-term weight loss goals and optimum wellness.

We hope you enjoy the cookbook and that we've introduced a wild splash of energy through healthy, revitalizing and amazingly tasty juicing recipes, carefully selected and nicely presented in it. You are offered a large choice of vegetable, fruit, berry, and herbal juices, all of which are rich in vitamins, phytonutrients, soluble fiber, and microelements, which are extremely important for keeping fit, energetic, and healthy. The book was aimed at helping you discover as many interesting combinations of various juices as possible so that your everyday juicing procedure is not restrained to just apples, carrots, or strawberries.

The next step is to purchase a great juicer and start trying out the recipes. Learn to value the process of juicing for it may be the best thing that has ever happened to your health.

Learning about juicing is just a baby step towards a healthier, happier life, but it makes all the difference. Understanding what juicing can do for you will only strengthen your commitment to yourself to start living healthy.

Drinking your fruits and vegetables can literally improve every aspect of your life. It will help you maintain a healthy weight, thereby boosting your confidence. It will give you the energy to overcome everyday demands. It will help you focus, think better, and sleep better. It will help you avoid many types of diseases. But most of all, juicing will make you feel happier and change the way you look at life. There is no more perfect time to make a health change than *now*. After all, none of us are getting any younger.

These recipes are sure to make a major change in your life, which you will notice from the very first week of starting your exciting adventure into the world of juicing. However, we strongly recommend that you follow the ingredient lists closely and do not overdo it with your daily intake of juices. A small cup of freshly squeezed juice may contain more calories than a whole meal. Therefore, you need to make sure you are ready to embark on an active lifestyle and make the best use of these healthy calories, using them for energy and not for a fat layer around the waistline.

Remember, if you continue an unhealthy lifestyle, no one will suffer the consequences later on but you. So, start today and keep juicing. Don't make juicing a habit; make it an integral part of your healthy, happy lifestyle.

Thank you and good luck!

Printed in Great Britain
by Amazon